Hepatology and Critical Care

Editors

RAHUL S. NANCHAL
RAM M. SUBRAMANIAN

CRITICAL CARE CLINICS

www.criticalcare.theclinics.com

Consulting Editor
RICHARD W. CARLSON

July 2016 • Volume 32 • Number 3

ELSEVIER

1600 John F. Kennedy Boulevard • Suite 1800 • Philadelphia, Pennsylvania, 19103-2899

http://www.theclinics.com

CRITICAL CARE CLINICS Volume 32, Number 3
July 2016 ISSN 0749-0704, ISBN-13: 978-0-323-44842-0

Editor: Patrick Manley
Developmental Editor: Casey Jackson

Critical Care Clinics (ISSN: 0749-0704) is published quarterly by Elsevier Inc., 360 Park Avenue South, New York, NY 10010-1710. Months of issue are January, April, July, and October. Business and Editorial Offices: 1600 John F. Kennedy Blvd., Suite 1800, Philadelphia, PA 19103-2899. Customer Service Office: 6277 Sea Harbor Drive, Orlando, FL 32887-4800. Periodicals postage paid at New York, NY and additional mailing offices. Subscription prices are $215.00 per year for US individuals, $551.00 per year for US institution, $100.00 per year for US students and residents, $255.00 per year for Canadian individuals, $691.00 per year for Canadian institutions, $300.00 per year for international individuals, $691.00 per year for international institutions and $150.00 per year for Canadian and foreign students/ residents. To receive student/resident rate, orders must be accompanied by name of affiliated institution, date of term, and the signature of program/residency coordinator on institution letterhead. Orders will be billed at individual rate until proof of status is received. Foreign air speed delivery is included in all *Clinics* subscription prices. All prices are subject to change without notice. POSTMASTER: Send address changes to *Critical Care Clinics*, Elsevier Periodicals Customer Service, 11830 Westline Industrial Drive, St. Louis, MO 63146. **Customer Service: 1-800-654-2452 (US). From outside of the US, call 1-314-447-8871. Fax: 1-314-447-8029. E-mail: journalscustomerservice-usa@ elsevier.com (for print support) or journalsonlinesupport-usa@elsevier.com (for online support).**

Reprints. For copies of 100 or more of articles in this publication, please contact the Commercial Reprints Department, Elsevier Inc., 360 Park Avenue South, New York, NY 10010-1710. Tel.: 212-633-3874; Fax: 212-633-3820; E-mail: reprints@elsevier.com.

Critical Care Clinics is also published in Spanish by Editorial Inter-Medica, Junin 917, 1er A, 1113, Buenos Aires, Argentina.

Critical Care Clinics is covered in *MEDLINE/PubMed (Index Medicus), EMBASE/Excerpta Medica, Current Concepts/ Clinical Medicine, ISI/BIOMED, and Chemical Abstracts.*

Contributors

CONSULTING EDITOR

RICHARD W. CARLSON, MD, PhD
Chairman Emeritus, Director, Medical Intensive Care Unit, Department of Medicine, Maricopa Medical Center; Professor, University of Arizona College of Medicine; Professor, Department of Medicine, Mayo Graduate School of Medicine, Phoenix, Arizona; Mayo Clinic, Scottsdale, Arizona

EDITORS

RAHUL S. NANCHAL, MD, MS, FCCM
Associate Professor of Medicine and Neurology, Director, Medical Intensive Care Unit, Director, Critical Care Fellowship Program, Division of Pulmonary and Critical Care Medicine, Froedtert and Medical College of Wisconsin, Milwaukee, Wisconsin

RAM M. SUBRAMANIAN, MD, FCCM
Associate Professor of Medicine and Surgery, Medical Director Liver Transplantation, Division of Hepatology and Critical Care Medicine, Emory University, Atlanta, Georgia

AUTHORS

SHAHRYAR AHMAD, MD
Fellow, Division of Pulmonary and Critical Care Medicine, Medical College of Wisconsin, Milwaukee, Wisconsin

MICHAEL G. ALLISON, MD
Attending Physician, Critical Care Medicine, St. Agnes Hospital, Baltimore, Maryland

SIKANDAR ANSARI, MD
Assistant Professor, Division of Pulmonary and Critical Care Medicine, Department of Medicine, Medical College of Wisconsin, Milwaukee, Wisconsin

ANNIE N. BIESBOER, PharmD, BCPS
Assistant Professor of Pharmacy Practice, Concordia University of Wisconsin School of Pharmacy, Mequon, Wisconsin

TESSA W. DAMM, DO
Critical Care Medicine and Neurocritical Care, Aurora Critical Care Service, Milwaukee, Wisconsin

MICAH FISHER, MD
Assistant Professor, Division of Pulmonary and Critical Care Medicine, Department of Medicine, Emory Clinic 'A', Atlanta, Georgia

JOLIE GALLAGHER, PharmD
PGY2 Critical Care Pharmacy Resident, Department of Pharmaceutical Services, Emory University Hospital; Adjunct Clinical Instructor, Mercer University College of Pharmacy, Atlanta, Georgia

STEVEN M. HOLLENBERG, MD
Professor of Medicine, Program Director, Department of Cardiovascular Disease, Cooper University Hospital, Camden, New Jersey

PREM A. KANDIAH, MD
Assistant Professor, Division of Neuro Critical Care, Department of Neurosurgery, Co-appointment in Surgical Critical Care, Emory University Hospital, Atlanta, Georgia

CONSTANTINE J. KARVELLAS, MD, SM, FRCPC
Associate Professor of Medicine, Divisions of Hepatology and Critical Care Medicine, University of Alberta, Edmonton, Alberta, Canada

MARK T. KEEGAN, MB, MRCPI, MSc
Professor, Division of Critical Care, Department of Anesthesiology, Mayo Clinic, Rochester, Minnesota

ALLEY J. KILLIAN, PharmD, BCPS
Clinical Pharmacy Specialist, Surgical Critical Care, Department of Pharmaceutical Services, Emory University Hospital, Atlanta, Georgia

DAVID J. KRAMER, MD, FACP
Medical Director, Aurora Critical Care Service, Milwaukee, Wisconsin; Clinical Professor of Medicine (Adjunct), University of Wisconsin, School of Medicine and Public Health, Madison, Wisconsin

GAGAN KUMAR, MD, MA
Intensivist, Department of Critical Care, Phoebe Putney Memorial Hospital, Albany, Georgia

RAHUL S. NANCHAL, MD, MS, FCCM
Associate Professor of Medicine and Neurology, Director, Medical Intensive Care Unit, Director, Critical Care Fellowship Program, Division of Pulmonary and Critical Care Medicine, Froedtert and Medical College of Wisconsin, Milwaukee, Wisconsin

JODY C. OLSON, MD
Assistant Professor of Medicine and Surgery, Hepatology and Critical Care Medicine, University of Kansas Medical Center, Kansas City, Kansas

VIJAYA S. RAMALINGAM, MD
Assistant Professor, Division of Pulmonary and Critical Care Medicine, Department of Medicine, Medical College of Wisconsin, Milwaukee, Wisconsin

KEVIN R. REGNER, MD, MS
Division of Nephrology, Medical College of Wisconsin, Milwaukee, Wisconsin

ASHUTOSH SACHDEVA, MBBS, FCCP
Assistant Professor of Medicine, Director, Interventional Pulmonary Program, Division of Pulmonary and Critical Care, University of Maryland School of Medicine, Baltimore, Maryland

KIA SAEIAN, MD, MSc Epi
Professor of Medicine-Gastroenterology, Medical College of Wisconsin, Milwaukee, Wisconsin

CARL B. SHANHOLTZ, MD
Professor of Medicine, Director, Medical Intensive Care Unit, Division of Pulmonary and Critical Care, University of Maryland School of Medicine, Baltimore, Maryland

KAI SINGBARTL, MD, MPH, FCCM
Department of Anesthesiology, Milton S. Hershey Medical Center, Penn State College of Medicine, Hershey, Pennsylvania

RAM M. SUBRAMANIAN, MD, FCCM
Associate Professor of Medicine and Surgery, Medical Director Liver Transplantation, Divisions of Hepatology and Critical Care Medicine, Emory University, Atlanta, Georgia

BRETT WALDMAN, MD
Clinical Fellow, Department of Cardiovascular Disease, Cooper University Hospital, Camden, New Jersey

Contents

> Chronic liver disease is the fifth leading cause of death worldwide and represents a major burden for the health care community. Cirrhosis is a progressive disease resulting in end-stage liver failure, which in the absence of liver transplantation is fatal. Acute-on-chronic liver failure carries high short-term mortality but is potentially reversible. Viral hepatitis, alcohol, and nonalcoholic fatty liver disease remain the principal causes of liver disease. Though treatments exist for hepatitis B and C, they remain unavailable to many with these diseases. This article reviews the epidemiology of advanced liver disease and the concept of acute-on-chronic liver failure.

> Hepatic encephalopathy occurs ubiquitously in all causes of advanced liver failure, however, its implications on mortality diverge and vary depending upon acuity and severity of liver failure. This associated mortality has decreased in subsets of liver failure over the last 20 years. Aside from liver transplantation, this improvement is not attributable to a single intervention but likely to a combination of practical advances in critical care management. Misconceptions surrounding many facets of hepatic encephalopathy exists due to heterogeneity in presentation, pathophysiology and outcome. This review is intended to highlight the important concepts, rationales and strategies for managing hepatic encephalopathy.

> In the cirrhotic liver, distortion of the normal liver architecture is caused by structural and vascular changes. Portal hypertension is often associated with a hyperdynamic circulatory syndrome in which cardiac output and heart rate are increased and systemic vascular resistance is decreased. The release of several vasoactive substances is the primary factor involved in the reduction of mesenteric arterial resistance, resulting in sodium and water retention with eventual formation of ascites. Management of these patients with acute cardiac dysfunction often requires invasive hemodynamic monitoring in an intensive care unit setting to tailor decisions regarding use of fluids and vasopressors.

> With the evolution of surgical and anesthetic techniques, liver transplantation has become "routine," allowing for modifications of practice to decrease perioperative complications and costs. There is debate over the necessity for intensive care unit admission for patients with satisfactory preoperative status and a smooth intraoperative course. Postoperative care is made easier when the liver graft performs optimally. Assessment of graft function, vigilance for complications after the major surgical insult, and optimization of multiple systems affected by liver disease are essential aspects of postoperative care. The intensivist plays a vital role in an integrated multidisciplinary transplant team.

CRITICAL CARE CLINICS

THE CLINICS ARE AVAILABLE ONLINE!
Access your subscription at:
www.theclinics.com

Preface

Hepato-centric Musings of Two Intensivists—Back to the Future

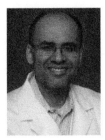 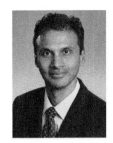

Rahul S. Nanchal, MD, MS, FCCM   Ram M. Subramanian, MD, FCCM
Editors

The liver as a structure has intrigued humans for perhaps more than 30 millennia. In the ancient world, it was regarded as "the seat of the soul." Galen viewed the body as hepato-centric and considered the liver the origin of veins and the source of blood. The punishment of Prometheus in Greek mythology (artistically depicted as *Prometheus Bound* [Philadelphia Museum of Art]) for stealing fire from the Gods to give to mankind was to have an eagle tear out and devour his liver each night, which grew back every morning for the process to be repeated. This connotes a remarkable familiarity with the extraordinary regenerative capabilities of the liver. From Hippocrates, who recognized the neuropsychiatric manifestations of advanced liver disease, Ludwig van Beethoven, who underwent repeated paracentesis and eventually succumbed to hepatic coma, Kiernan's description of the hexagonal hepatic lobule, illustrations of Mallory bodies by Frank Burr Mallory in the hepatocytes of patients with alcoholic liver disease, William Bennett Bean's extensive narratives of vascular spiders, to Roberto Groszmann's remarkable insights into the hyperdynamic circulation of liver disease, the literature is rife with a woven tapestry of gradually accumulating evidence that has led to the modern view of liver disease and its complex and fascinating cross-talk with every organ in the body. We stand on the shoulders of giants, and not everyone is acknowledged in this short preface; they are too numerous to tally. Their collective wisdom and seminal observations of the past have paved the way for the present, and more importantly, placed us on the cusp of an incredibly bright future of discovery and therapeutics.

Everyone has a favorite organ; ours is the liver. Two intensivists believe that the liver, often forgotten and frequently neglected, is a master orchestrator of outcomes from critical illness. This is particularly true if the liver is ailing, perhaps more so than any other organ of the body. In this issue, we endeavor to provide the reader with a broad landscape of the far-reaching consequences of hepatic failure on distant organ function, the intricacies of the cross-talk between the liver and multiple organs, and the

Crit Care Clin 32 (2016) xiii–xiv
http://dx.doi.org/10.1016/j.ccc.2016.04.001
0749-0704/16/$ – see front matter © 2016 Published by Elsevier Inc.

evolution of paradigms of care for the critically ill patient with liver disease. As we reminisce about our chosen path from when seasoned clinicians taught us to recognize the subtle and not so subtle signs of liver disease to the current era of advances in liver support and transplantation, we fondly and joyfully acknowledge the eminent role of our children, Avi, Sanath, and Saurav, in our passions and successes. We are truly back to the future!

Rahul S. Nanchal, MD, MS, FCCM
Division of Pulmonary and Critical Care Medicine
Froedtert and Medical College of Wisconsin
9200 West Wisconsin Avenue, Suite E5200
Milwaukee, WI 53226, USA

Ram M. Subramanian, MD, FCCM
Emory University
1365 Clifton Road
Building B 6100
Atlanta, GA 30322, USA

E-mail addresses:
rnanchal@mcw.edu (R.S. Nanchal)
rmsubra@emory.edu (R.M. Subramanian)

Acute-on-chronic and Decompensated Chronic Liver Failure

Definitions, Epidemiology, and Prognostication

Jody C. Olson, MD

KEYWORDS

- Cirrhosis • Acute-on-chronic liver failure (ACLF) • Transplantation
- Advanced liver disease

KEY POINTS

- Chronic liver disease is the fifth leading cause of death worldwide.
- Advanced liver disease results in multisystem organ failure and is responsible for a significant intensive care burden. Major causes of liver disease are viral hepatitis, alcohol, and nonalcoholic fatty liver disease.
- Advances in treatment of viral infections may change the epidemiology of liver disease in the future; however, at the present time the incidence of cirrhosis is continuing to increase.
- Cirrhosis is a progressive disease in most cases and results in death in the absence of transplant.
- Acute-on-chronic liver failure is a unique clinical entity that differs from cirrhosis in that it is potentially reversible.

INTRODUCTION

Strictly defined, cirrhosis is the "histological development of regenerative nodules surrounded by fibrous bands in response to chronic liver injury."[1] Chronic pathologic processes that result in cirrhosis include chronic viral infections, excess alcohol use, nonalcoholic fatty liver disease (NAFLD), autoimmune diseases, genetic diseases of copper and iron metabolism, alpha1-antitrypsin deficiency, and biliary obstruction. Regardless of the type of liver insult, ongoing inflammation results in chronic liver disease via two distinct, but closely related, pathologic processes. First, chronic inflammation leads to activation of hepatic stellate cells, which are the key fibrogenic effector cells within the liver. Activation of stellate cells results in deposition of fibrous

Hepatology and Critical Care Medicine, University of Kansas Medical Center, 3901 Rainbow Boulevard, MS 1023, Kansas City, KS 66160, USA
E-mail address: jolson2@kumc.edu

Crit Care Clin 32 (2016) 301–309
http://dx.doi.org/10.1016/j.ccc.2016.02.001
0749-0704/16/$ – see front matter © 2016 Elsevier Inc. All rights reserved.

connective tissue throughout the liver.[2] The progressive deposition of fibrous connective tissue leads to severe disruption of both the vascular and microscopic lobular architecture of the liver, leading to portal hypertension. Second, with progressive fibrosis and ongoing hepatocyte injury, extinction of hepatocytes occurs, resulting in a decrease in the functional metabolic capacity of the liver.

As an aside, it is important to recognize that liver cell death does not necessarily equate to chronic liver disease. For example, acute liver failure that results from toxin exposure, such as acetaminophen, may result in catastrophic death of hepatocytes and resultant liver failure. Patients may fully recover from episodes of acute liver failure; recovery is typically complete and does not result in chronic liver disease. In this article, advanced liver disease refers to chronic liver disease and cirrhosis, and specifically excludes acute liver failure, which is a separate clinical entity with an entirely different epidemiology and approach to management.

From a more practical standpoint, cirrhosis must be understood as a spectrum of disease and is a heterogeneous disorder; cirrhosis is not an all-or-none phenomenon. Patients with early cirrhosis may have no clinical or biochemical manifestations of liver disease, whereas those with advanced-stage cirrhosis often present with multisystem organ failure. Liver fibrosis is progressive in the vast majority of cases; however, with the advent of improved therapies for many diseases, such as curative therapy for chronic hepatitis C infection, clinicians now appreciate that fibrosis may be arrested, and in some cases may be reversible.[3]

CAUSES AND RISK FACTORS FOR DEVELOPMENT OF CIRRHOSIS
Viral Disease

Hepatitis B is a DNA virus responsible for development of both acute and chronic liver disease; worldwide it affects between 350 million and 400 million people and is responsible for liver-related deaths in 1 million people annually.[4] Hepatitis C virus is an RNA virus infecting 3% of the world population, with high prevalence in the Middle East, Asia, and northern Africa.[5] There are an estimated 3 million people infected with hepatitis C in the United States alone, with half of those having undiagnosed disease.[6] Improved antiviral therapies have resulted in treatments that may dramatically alter the course of these diseases. Hepatitis B may be controlled, with a low incidence of development of viral resistance. Hepatitis C is now curable in most infected patients with vastly simplified regimens. However, the very high cost of antiviral therapies renders them unobtainable for most infected individuals across the globe at the present time. Further complicating the issue is that millions remain undiagnosed, thereby preventing initiation of appropriate therapy. Thus, in spite of dramatic advances in treatment, viral hepatitis will remain a major contributor to the development of cirrhosis for the foreseeable future.

Alcohol misuse is a major risk factor in the development of chronic liver disease worldwide[7] and is the main risk factor for the development of cirrhosis in Europe.[8] In general, there is a dose-response relationship between the amount and duration of alcohol consumption and development of cirrhosis. However, only 15% to 35% of heavy drinkers develop cirrhosis,[9,10] thus indicating that additional influences are involved in the development of alcoholic liver disease. In addition to genetic influences, previous studies have identified additional risk factors that, when present, increase the chance of developing cirrhosis caused by alcohol. These risk factors include female sex, obesity, smoking, and chronic hepatitis C infection.[11,12] A recent study by Askgaard and colleagues[13] evaluated patterns of alcohol consumption as a risk factor for development of cirrhosis. Daily drinking in men conferred a hazard ratio of 3.65 (95% confidence interval, 2.39–5.55) compared with drinking only 2 to 4 days per week.

It is generally accepted that NAFLD is the most common chronic liver condition in the world. NAFLD encompasses hepatic steatosis without evidence of liver inflammation and nonalcoholic steatohepatitis (NASH). NASH is a more pathogenic form of NAFLD and leads to the development of fibrosis and cirrhosis.[14] Reported prevalence of NAFLD varies widely depending on the population studied and the methods used to assess this liver disorder (eg, biopsy vs noninvasive imaging). A 2011 systematic review by Vernon and colleagues[15] reported the prevalence of NAFLD in the United States at 30% with median worldwide prevalence of 20%. The increasing incidences of NAFLD and NASH mirror worldwide trends in obesity and the metabolic syndrome.[16] At present, NASH is the third leading cause for liver transplant in the United States and, if the current trajectory continues, it is likely to become the most common.[17]

In addition to the major risk factors for development of cirrhosis listed earlier, many other disease states result in cirrhosis of the liver.

Metabolic Disease

Hereditary hemochromatosis is a disease of iron overload and is the most common genetic disorder affecting white people with a prevalence of 1 in 220 to 250 persons.[18] Wilson disease is an autosomal recessive disorder of copper metabolism affecting 1 in 30,000 persons worldwide.[19] Both conditions may result in the development of cirrhosis in the absence of proper treatment. In contrast with hereditary hemochromatosis, Wilson disease may present as acute or chronic liver failure.

Autoimmune Disease

Several autoimmune conditions lead to advanced liver disease. Primary sclerosing cholangitis (PSC) is a disease of the intrahepatic and extrahepatic bile ducts that results in progressive biliary stricturing and may be complicated by development of cirrhosis and cholangiocarcinoma. Although thought to be immune mediated, the exact mechanism for disease development has not been fully elucidated.[20] PSC has no known treatment.

Primary biliary cirrhosis (PBC) is also a progressive cholestatic disease of the bile ducts (primarily intrahepatic). PBC carries a highly specific autoimmune profile with 90% to 95% of patients having positive serologies for antimitochondrial antibodies, with less than 1% of healthy controls being positive.[21] PBC does respond to treatment with ursodeoxycholic acid, which delays histologic progression of biliary disease and improves transplant-free survival.[22,23]

Autoimmune hepatitis, as the name implies, results from a T cell–mediated attack directed against liver antigens with resultant inflammation and fibrosis, and frequently responds to immune-modulating therapies. The natural history of autoimmune hepatitis varies greatly from cases of acute liver failure to essentially asymptomatic disease.[24] Other less common causes of advanced liver disease are listed in **Box 1**.

EPIDEMIOLOGY OF ADVANCED LIVER DISEASE

Advanced liver disease presents a significant global health burden. Worldwide, cirrhosis is the 12th leading cause of death, representing more than 1 million deaths in 2012.[25] However, when deaths attributed to viral hepatitis (B and C) are added to liver cancer (which occurs largely secondary to cirrhosis and/or viral hepatitis), advanced liver disease becomes the fifth leading cause of death worldwide (**Fig. 1**), responsible for nearly 2 million deaths annually.[25]

Box 1
Causes of advanced liver disease

Most common:
- Chronic hepatitis C infection
- Chronic hepatitis B infection
- Alcohol
- NASH

Less common:
- Wilson disease
- Primary sclerosing cholangitis
- Primary biliary cirrhosis
- Alpha1-antitrypsin deficiency
- Autoimmune hepatitis
- Hereditary hemochromatosis

Rare:
- Glycogen storage disease
- Methotrexate
- Amiodarone
- Heart failure
- Schistosomiasis

A recent study published by Scaglione and colleagues[26] examined the prevalence of cirrhosis in the United States using the National Health and Nutrition Examination Survey data from 1999 to 2010. The prevalence of cirrhosis in the United States is estimated to be 0.27%, which corresponds with slightly more than 630,000 adults.[26] A startling finding in this study was that nearly 70% of patients identified as potentially having cirrhosis could not recall being diagnosed with liver disease,[26] thus indicating that this disease with high prevalence remains grossly under-recognized.

According to the United States Centers for Disease Control (CDC) mortality data for deaths attributed to cirrhosis, cirrhosis is the 12th leading cause of death overall.[27] When analyzed in the context of distinct age groups, liver disease ranks as the seventh leading cause of death in adults aged 25 to 44 years, and the fifth leading cause of death in adults aged 45 to 64 years.[27] However, the CDC data are flawed as they rely on a narrow definition for the identification of liver disease. CDC estimates are based only on death certificate data which lists as a cause of death; alcoholic liver disease, chronic hepatitis, and fibrosis and cirrhosis of the liver. This method clearly fails to identify many cirrhosis associated deaths.[27] Recognizing the flaws in the CDC data,

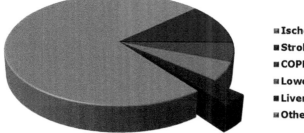

Ischemic Heart Disease
Stroke
COPD
Lower Resp Infections
Liver Disease
Other

Fig. 1. Top worldwide causes of death: the worldwide burden of liver disease. Deaths attributed to liver disease include deaths caused by viral hepatitis B and C, and liver cancer. COPD, chronic obstructive pulmonary disease; Resp, respiratory.

Asrani and colleagues[28] provided a more comprehensive assessment of the true liver-related mortality in the United States in a 2013 study. In this study, Mayo Clinic researchers used expanded criteria to identify deaths directly attributable to advanced liver disease. In addition to the definition used by the CDC, the Mayo group added the following other liver diagnoses: hepatic failure, unspecified; fatty change of the liver; hepatorenal syndrome; liver disease, unspecified; chronic hepatitis B and C; acute hepatitis B; and hepatobiliary cancer.[28] By applying expanded criteria, the Mayo team estimated that the 2008 death rate caused by advanced liver disease was 66,007; more than double the CDC estimate of 29,921.[28] An additional strength of the Asrani[28] study was the comparison of clinical data from the Rochester Epidemiology Project,[29] which served to verify the purely administrative data in the CDC report.

Given the significant morbidity associated with cirrhosis, it is no surprise that advanced liver disease is responsible for a substantial number of intensive care unit (ICU) admissions. It has previously been estimated that there are in excess of 26,000 ICU admissions related to cirrhosis annually, with an in-hospital mortality of greater than 50%.[30] The average cost of an admission is roughly $116,000 and an estimated $3 billion in annual charges are associated with the ICU care of patients with advanced liver disease.[30] Moreover, although ICU admissions with many chronic conditions have decreased over time, ICU admissions related to cirrhosis have remained unchanged (data not published, Kim W. Ray, MD, 2008).

CLINICAL IMPLICATIONS OF ADVANCED LIVER DISEASE: ACUTE-ON-CHRONIC VERSUS DECOMPENSATED CHRONIC LIVER DISEASE

The natural history of advanced liver disease provides that the disease may be broadly grouped into 2 categories: compensated and decompensated states. In compensated cirrhosis, manifestations of disease are minimal. The transition to decompensated disease occurs when symptoms of cirrhosis manifest in overt symptoms because of progressive architectural disruption and decreasing functional capacity of the liver. The principal events that signify a transition to decompensated disease are the development of esophageal varices, hepatic encephalopathy, or ascites. The transition from compensated disease to a decompensated state occurs at a rate of 5% to 7% per year[31] and has important prognostic implications. Median survival in patients with compensated disease is 12 years and decreases to 2 years after decompensation ensues.[31] Accumulation of decompensating events also worsens prognosis; for example, a patient who has upper gastrointestinal bleeding alone has an estimated 5-year mortality of 20%, but this increases to 88% after the development of a second decompensating event, such as the development of ascites after a variceal hemorrhage.[32] Liver transplant remains the only curative option for advanced decompensated cirrhosis. However, in many parts of the world, transplants are not available, and, in countries where transplants are available, demand for organs far exceeds supply. It is for these reasons that advanced cirrhosis is a terminal disease for most patients with this condition. The Model for End-stage Liver Disease (MELD) score has been extensively validated as a tool to predict short-term (90-day) mortality in patients with advanced liver disease[33] (Fig. 2). The MELD score is now used in many countries to prioritize patients on liver transplant waiting lists, thereby giving highest priority to patients at the highest risk for short-term mortality.

In addition to the primary manifestations of cirrhosis noted earlier, decompensated liver disease affects virtually all organ systems. Examples include disorders of renal function, such as abnormalities in fluid handling and overt renal failure (eg, hepatorenal

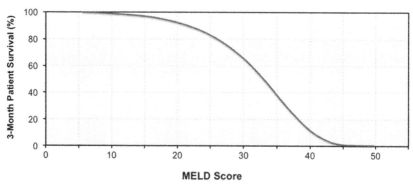

Fig. 2. 90 day mortality as a function of MELD score.

syndrome); gastrointestinal issues such as malnutrition, and motility disturbances; cardiac dysfunction with hyperdynamic circulation and systemic hypotension; endocrine abnormalities resulting in abnormal sodium handling, gynecomastia, osteoporosis, and glucose dysregulation; and pulmonary disorders, including portopulmonary hypertension and hepatopulmonary syndrome. All patients with cirrhosis are at risk for development of hepatocellular carcinoma, although rates are highest in patients with viral hepatitis, who develop hepatocellular carcinoma at rates of 3% to 8% per year.[34] When identified early, hepatocellular carcinoma is a treatable disease and may be cured with resection or liver transplant. Because of the complex interactions between the liver and all other organ systems, patients with cirrhosis who become critically ill provide distinct challenges for critical care teams.

The last decade has seen a growing interest in the concept of acute-on-chronic liver failure (ACLF) as a unique clinical entity that occurs in patients with chronic liver disease. In brief, ACLF is recognized as an acute deterioration of liver function occurring in patients with compensated or stably decompensated liver disease.[35,36] This phenomenon is frequently associated with a precipitating event (eg, infection or acute variceal hemorrhage) and results in multisystem organ failure, the need for intensive care support, and carries a high short-term mortality.[37] In contrast with the natural progression of advanced cirrhosis, which in the absence of transplant is eventually fatal, ACLF when identified and acted on early may carry an element of reversibility (**Fig. 3**). For these reasons, advancing the understanding of the concept of ACLF is particularly important for intensivists caring for patients with cirrhosis in the ICU as it may serve to guide decisions with regard to application of medical therapies and help identify cases in which further aggressive care is futile. Previously ACLF was largely a theoretic framework that lacked a foundation in evidence. However, recent work published by the European Association for the Study of Liver Disease–Chronic Liver Failure Consortium (EASL-CLIF) now gives a more evidence-based and pragmatic description of ACLF and provides a framework to aid in prognosis of these gravely ill patients.[38] Although work by the EASL-CLIF consortium has continued to significantly advance the understanding of ACLF, differentiating ACLF from true end-stage cirrhosis remains difficult because there is no single sign or test that identifies this entity and therefore practical application of this important concept by general intensivists remains a formidable challenge.

DISCUSSION

Advanced liver disease is responsible for a significant worldwide health burden. Advances in treatment of viral hepatitis may decrease the overall disease burden of

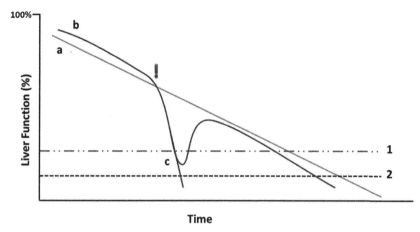

Fig. 3. The concept of acute-on-chronic liver failure. (*a*) The natural progression of chronic liver disease with decreasing functional capacity of the liver as a function of time. (*b*) Acute-on-chronic liver failure; at the point indicated by an exclamation mark the patient has a secondary insult (eg, acute bacterial infection) resulting in rapid decline of liver function. (*c*) The critical point for recovery; with appropriate intervention a patient may recover and return to a compensated state. If improvement does not occur, patients will die, which occurs in roughly 50% of cases. Lines 1 and 2 are arbitrarily drawn at points to represent the threshold for decompensation (organ failures) (*1*) and death (*2*).

advanced liver disease in the future; however, at present these therapies are not widely available because of extreme cost. The incidence of nonalcoholic liver disease is also increasing, thus the worldwide incidence of cirrhosis is likely to continue to increase for the foreseeable future. Patients with advanced liver disease experience extensive medical complications and have a high rate of hospitalization combined with frequent admissions to the ICU. This patient population provides distinct challenges for intensivists. Treatment options for patients with advanced liver disease are mainly supportive, with the only definitive treatment option being liver transplant. Those in need of life-saving liver transplant far outnumber organ availability.

Differentiating which patients are truly end stage and thus unlikely to benefit from aggressive life support from those who have ACLF remains difficult. All patients who present to the ICU in the setting of advanced liver disease deserve consultation with transplant specialists to determine whether transplant is a potential option. In the absence of a viable transplant option and in patients in whom ongoing aggressive life support has failed to improve the overall condition, the prognosis is dismal. In order to obtain the best outcomes for this difficult population, teams consisting of specialists in critical care and hepatology are required.

REFERENCES

1. Schuppan D, Afdhal NH. Liver cirrhosis. Lancet 2008;371(9615):838–51.
2. Pinzani M. Pathophysiology of liver fibrosis. Dig Dis 2015;33(4):492–7.
3. Povero D, Busletta C, Novo E, et al. Liver fibrosis: a dynamic and potentially reversible process. Histol Histopathol 2010;25(8):1075–91.
4. Dienstag JL. Hepatitis B virus infection. N Engl J Med 2008;359(14):1486–500.
5. Feeney ER, Chung RT. Antiviral treatment of hepatitis C. BMJ 2014;348:g3308.
6. Holmberg SD, Spradling PR, Moorman AC, et al. Hepatitis C in the United States. N Engl J Med 2013;368(20):1859–61.

7. Rehm J, Mathers C, Popova S, et al. Global burden of disease and injury and economic cost attributable to alcohol use and alcohol-use disorders. Lancet 2009;373(9682):2223–33.

8. Zatonski WA, Sulkowska U, Manczuk M, et al. Liver cirrhosis mortality in Europe, with special attention to Central and Eastern Europe. Eur Addict Res 2010;16(4): 193–201.

9. European Association for the Study of Liver. EASL clinical practical guidelines: management of alcoholic liver disease. J Hepatol 2012;57(2):399–420.

10. McCullough AJ, O'Shea RS, Dasarathy S. Diagnosis and management of alcoholic liver disease. J Dig Dis 2011;12(4):257–62.

11. Dam MK, Flensborg-Madsen T, Eliasen M, et al. Smoking and risk of liver cirrhosis: a population-based cohort study. Scand J Gastroenterol 2013;48(5): 585–91.

12. Torres DM, Williams CD, Harrison SA. Features, diagnosis, and treatment of nonalcoholic fatty liver disease. Clin Gastroenterol Hepatol 2012;10(8):837–58.

13. Askgaard G, Gronbaek M, Kjaer MS, et al. Alcohol drinking pattern and risk of alcoholic liver cirrhosis: a prospective cohort study. J Hepatol 2015;62(5):1061–7.

14. Tilg H, Moschen AR. Evolution of inflammation in nonalcoholic fatty liver disease: the multiple parallel hits hypothesis. Hepatology 2010;52(5):1836–46.

15. Vernon G, Baranova A, Younossi ZM. Systematic review: the epidemiology and natural history of non-alcoholic fatty liver disease and non-alcoholic steatohepatitis in adults. Aliment Pharmacol Ther 2011;34(3):274–85.

16. Chalasani N, Younossi Z, Lavine JE, et al. The diagnosis and management of non-alcoholic fatty liver disease: practice guideline by the American Association for the Study of Liver Diseases, American College of Gastroenterology, and the American Gastroenterological Association. Hepatology 2012;55(6):2005–23.

17. Charlton MR, Burns JM, Pedersen RA, et al. Frequency and outcomes of liver transplantation for nonalcoholic steatohepatitis in the United States. Gastroenterology 2011;141(4):1249–53.

18. Bacon BR, Adams PC, Kowdley KV, et al. Diagnosis and management of hemochromatosis: 2011 practice guideline by the American Association for the Study of Liver Diseases. Hepatology 2011;54(1):328–43.

19. Mak CM, Lam CW. Diagnosis of Wilson's disease: a comprehensive review. Crit Rev Clin Lab Sci 2008;45(3):263–90.

20. Maggs JR, Chapman RW. An update on primary sclerosing cholangitis. Curr Opin Gastroenterol 2008;24(3):377–83.

21. Gershwin ME, Mackay IR, Sturgess A, et al. Identification and specificity of a cDNA encoding the 70 kd mitochondrial antigen recognized in primary biliary cirrhosis. J Immunol 1987;138(10):3525–31.

22. Lindor KD, Gershwin ME, Poupon R, et al. Primary biliary cirrhosis. Hepatology 2009;50(1):291–308.

23. Poupon RE, Lindor KD, Pares A, et al. Combined analysis of the effect of treatment with ursodeoxycholic acid on histologic progression in primary biliary cirrhosis. J Hepatol 2003;39(1):12–6.

24. Manns MP, Czaja AJ, Gorham JD, et al. Diagnosis and management of autoimmune hepatitis. Hepatology 2010;51(6):2193–213.

25. World Health Organization global health estimates for cause specific mortality 2014. Available at: http://www.who.int/healthinfo/global_burden_disease/estimates/en/index1.html. Accessed October 1, 2015.

26. Scaglione S, Kliethermes S, Cao G, et al. The epidemiology of cirrhosis in the United States: a population-based study. J Clin Gastroenterol 2015;49(8):690–6.

27. Heron M. Deaths: leading causes for 2012. Natl Vital Stat Rep 2015;64(10):1–94.
28. Asrani SK, Larson JJ, Yawn B, et al. Underestimation of liver-related mortality in the United States. Gastroenterology 2013;145(2):375–82.e1-2.
29. Melton LJ 3rd. History of the Rochester Epidemiology Project. Mayo Clin Proc 1996;71(3):266–74.
30. Olson JC, Wendon JA, Kramer DJ, et al. Intensive care of the patient with cirrhosis. Hepatology 2011;54(5):1864–72.
31. D'Amico G, Garcia-Tsao G, Pagliaro L. Natural history and prognostic indicators of survival in cirrhosis: a systematic review of 118 studies. J Hepatol 2006;44(1):217–31.
32. D'Amico G, Pasta L, Morabito A, et al. Competing risks and prognostic stages of cirrhosis: a 25-year inception cohort study of 494 patients. Aliment Pharmacol Ther 2014;39(10):1180–93.
33. Kamath PS, Wiesner RH, Malinchoc M, et al. A model to predict survival in patients with end-stage liver disease. Hepatology 2001;33(2):464–70.
34. Bruix J, Sherman M. Management of hepatocellular carcinoma: an update. Hepatology 2011;53(3):1020–2.
35. Jalan R, Gines P, Olson JC, et al. Acute-on chronic liver failure. J Hepatol 2012;57(6):1336–48.
36. Olson JC, Kamath PS. Acute-on-chronic liver failure: concept, natural history, and prognosis. Curr Opin Crit Care 2011;17(2):165–9.
37. Olson JC, Kamath PS. Acute-on-chronic liver failure: what are the implications? Curr Gastroenterol Rep 2012;14(1):63–6.
38. Gustot T, Fernandez J, Garcia E, et al. Clinical course of acute-on-chronic liver failure syndrome and effects on prognosis. Hepatology 2015;62(1):243–52.

Hepatic Encephalopathy— the Old and the New

Prem A. Kandiah, MD[a],*, Gagan Kumar, MD, MA[b]

KEYWORDS

- Hepatic encephalopathy • Acute liver failure • Fulminant hepatic failure
- Chronic liver failure • Acute-on-chronic liver failure

KEY POINTS

- An elevated plasma ammonia level (>150 µmol/L) in acute liver failure increases the risk of intracranial hypertension; however, a low level (<146 µmol/L) does not preclude it when associated with multiorgan failure.
- Acute-on-chronic liver failure patients admitted with overt hepatic encephalopathy have a significantly higher short-term mortality rate and small but devastating risk of brain herniation (4%) and are at an increased risk of intracranial hemorrhage (16%).
- Brain MRI pattern of restricted diffusion (cytotoxic edema) in hyperammonemia associated with urea cycle disorder or liver failure correlates in severity with plasma ammonia levels and clinical outcome.
- Therapeutic hypothermia is safe but does not confer a clear mortality benefit in acute liver failure.
- Invasive intracranial pressure monitoring used in an estimate of 20% to 30% of patients with acute liver failure in North America yields a 2.5% to 10% risk of intracranial hemorrhage with unproven benefit.
- Molecular adsorbent recirculating system and embolization of large spontaneous portosystemic shunting may facilitate improvement in grade of hepatic encephalopathy safely but without a proven mortality benefit.

INTRODUCTION

Hepatic encephalopathy (HE) represents brain dysfunction directly caused by liver insufficiency or portosystemic shunting (PSS) that manifests as a wide spectrum of neurologic and psychiatric deficits ranging from subclinical deficits to coma.

No commercial or financial conflict of interest and funding.

[a] Division of Neuro Critical Care, Department of Neurosurgery, Co-appointment in Surgical Critical Care, Emory University Hospital, 1364 Clifton Road Northeast, 2nd Floor, 2D ICU-D264, Atlanta, GA 30322, USA; [b] Department of Critical Care, Phoebe Putney Memorial Hospital, 417 Third Avenue, Albany, GA 31701, USA

* Corresponding author.

E-mail address: prem.kandiah@emoryhealthcare.org

CLASSIFICATION OF HEPATIC ENCEPHALOPATHY

To capture the complexity and breadth of HE, the recent 2014 combined European Association of the Study of the Liver and the American Association for the Study of Liver Diseases guidelines have integrated 4 characteristic factors into the classification of HE (**Table 1**): (1) underlying disease, (2) severity of manifestation, (3) time course, and (4) precipitating factors. Severity of manifestation was adapted from West Haven criteria[1] and merged with 3 newer definitions, minimal HE, covert HE, and overt HE. For the purpose of this critical care review, the focus is limited on overt HE (types A and C).

Table 1
Classification and grading of hepatic encephalopathy[a]

Classification of HE	Subclassification of HE	Defining Feature and Description	
1. Underlying disease[a]	Type A	Acute Liver Failure	
	Type B	Portal-systemic Bypass without intrinsic hepato-cellular damage	
	Type C	Cirrhosis and portal hypertension with portal-systemic shunts	
2. Severity of Manifestation[b]	Grade 0	No HE	No HE
		Psychometric or neuropsychological alterations without clinical evidence of mental change	Minimal HE or covert
	Grade I	Trivial lack of awareness Euphoria or anxiety Shortened attention span Impairment of addition or subtraction Altered sleep rhythm	Covert
	Grade II	Lethargy or apathy Disorientation for time Obvious personality change Inappropriate behavior Dyspraxia Asterixis	Overt
	Grade III	Somnolence to semistupor Responsive to stimuli Confused Gross disorientation Bizarre behavior	
	Grade IV	Coma	
3. Time course of presentation	Episodic	Single or episodes occurring >6 mo	
	Recurrent	Episodes occur <6 mo	
	Persistent	Behavioral alterations that are always present and interspersed with relapses of overt HE.	
4. Precipitating factors	None	—	
	Precipitated	Precipitating factors can be identified in nearly all bouts of episodic HE type C and should be actively sought and treated when found	

[a] European Association of the Study of the Liver and the American Association for the Study of Liver Diseases Hepatic encephalopathy Guidelines.[2]
[b] *Adapted from* Ferenci P, Lockwood A, Mullen K, et al. Hepatic encephalopathy–definition, nomenclature, diagnosis, and quantification: final report of the working party at the 11th World Congresses of Gastroenterology, Vienna, 1998. Hepatology 2002;35(3):716–21.

HEPATIC ENCEPHALOPATHY, CEREBRAL EDEMA, AND MORTALITY IN ACUTE LIVER FAILURE AND OVERT TYPE C HEPATIC ENCEPHALOPATHY

Cerebral edema (CE) at the cellular level (cytotoxic edema) or interstitial level (vasogenic edema) is a pathophysiologic hallmark of HE in acute and chronic liver failure. In chronic liver failure, the occurrence of CE is not apparent on a macroscopic level. Hence, the edema is not visible on conventional brain imaging, posing no concerns for elevated intracranial pressure (ICP).

Acute liver failure (ALF) is a devastating disease with mortality up to 40% to 50% caused by progressive multiorgan failure. Grade IV HE precedes the development of cerebral edema and intracranial hypertension (IH) culminating in transtentorial herniation. Historically the progression from HE to transtentorial herniation accounted for up to 75% to 80% of deaths in ALF.[3] With improved ICU care focusing on neuroprotective interventions, the mortality attributable to IH is in the range of 10% to 20%.[4]

Despite the absence of IH, the diagnosis of HE in chronic liver failure is associated with a 50% mortality rate at 1 year. The correlation between type C HE and increased mortality in cirrhosis has been difficult to decipher with the heterogeneity in overlapping multiorgan failure. The term *acute-on-chronic liver failure* (ACLF) more accurately captures the subgroup of chronic liver failure presenting with multiorgan failure. HE associated with ACLF has a significantly higher mortality rate compared with patients with decompensated cirrhosis[5] and, therefore, warrants early transfer to the ICU.

Unlike ALF, IH does not occur in decompensated cirrhosis but is infrequently reported in ACLF.[6,7] The rare occurrence of IH in ACLF is predicated on the acuity of the liver injury rather than the chronicity of the liver disease.[8] A more recent retrospective study noted that IH with death from tonsillar herniation was observed in 4% (3 of 48) of patients with ACLF.[9]

CLINICAL FEATURES AND APPROACH TO EVALUATING A PATIENT WITH HEPATIC ENCEPHALOPATHY

HE is a diagnosis of exclusion that should be probed with a detailed history, physical examination, laboratory investigation, and brain imaging. If the mental status decline of HE (grade 1–4) is witnessed with typical features and a precipitant identified, extensive workup for an alternate etiology is less imperative.

NEUROLOGIC ASSESSMENT IN OVERT HEPATIC ENCEPHALOPATHY

In addition to assessing orientation and attention (serial subtraction test) in West Heaven (WH) grade I to II HE, grading asterixis over 30 seconds is a quick and objective way to monitor progression of HE (**Table 2**).[10]

In more severe grades of HE, using the Glasgow Coma Scale allows a more refined discrimination of advanced grades of HE (**Table 3**). A traditional neurologic examination will frequently detect false localizing signs in severe HE including transient pupillary dysfunction, disconjugate gaze, gaze deviation, ocular bobbing, decorticate and decerebrate posturing, hyperreflexia, and up-going plantar reflexes, which may result in additional neuroimaging for reassurance. These findings are usually transient and resolve or shift in laterality within hours and can occasionally mimic the presentation of acute stroke or transient ischemic attack.

In ALF, pupillary light reaction frequently progresses from normal to hyperresponsive in early in WH grade II to III HE and subsequently hyporesponsive in WH

Table 2
Grading asterixsis to monitor progression of hepatic encephalopathy

Grade of Asterixis	Description[a]	Number of Flaps/30 s
Grade 0	No flapping motions	0
Grade I	Rare flapping motion	1–2
Grade II	Occasional, irregular flaps	3–4
Grade III	Frequent flaps	5–30

[a] Asterixis should be differentiated from fine and coarse tremor.
From Conn HBJ. Quantifying the severity of hepatic encephalopathy. Bloomington (IL): Medi-Ed Press; 1994.

grade IV.[11] Loss of pupillary function can signify brain herniation owing to uncal compression of ciliary fibers of cranial nerve III. However, loss of pupillary function may be caused by metabolic abnormality in late stages of HE. Despite this false-positive finding, close monitoring of pupils is critical in ALF, as reversal of brain herniation using osmotherapy is possible if detected immediately.

OBJECTIVES OF SERIAL LABORATORY TESTING RELEVANT TO HEPATIC ENCEPHALOPATHY AND INTRACRANIAL HYPERTENSION IN ACUTE LIVER FAILURE

1. Assessing onset, severity, and recovery of acute liver failure that parallels the onset and cessation of risk of IH development
2. Guiding management of cerebral edema by (1) monitoring plasma sodium levels, osmolarity, pH, CO_2, and plasma ammonia levels; (2) correcting hyponatremia, severe acidosis, and hypercarbia; and (3) augmenting plasma sodium levels and osmolality
3. Monitoring other end-organ function, detection of infection, and augmenting hemodynamic assessment

RISK FACTOR FOR DEVELOPMENT OF INTRACRANIAL HYPERTENSION IN ACUTE LIVER FAILURE

Plasma ammonia level of more than 150 to 200 μmol/L is a well-known risk factor for IH in ALF. More recently, Kitzberger and colleagues[12] reported that 25% of ALF patients had IH despite low plasma ammonia levels (NH3 <146 μmol/L). The disproportionately higher extracerebral severity of organ failure (SOFA) score in these patients emphasizes the substantial role of inflammation and organ failure in the development of cerebral hyperemia and diffuse cerebral edema. Assessment of risk factors for IH allows for further risk stratification and early intervention to prevent IH. A list of reported risk factors specific to ALF are listed in **Table 4**.

Table 3
Comparable Glasgow Coma Scale to Modified West Haven

West Haven Criteria Grade	Glasgow Coma Scale
I	14–15
II	12–15
III	7–12
IV	<7

Adapted from Bernal W, Wendon J. Acute liver failure. N Engl J Med 2013;369:2525–34.

Table 4	
Risk Factors associated with intracranial hypertension in ALF	
Risk Factors of IH	**Possible Mechanisms and Rationale**
1. Meets Kings College Criteria	Correlates with severity of liver injury resulting in cerebral hyperemia caused by severe inflammation
2. Plasma ammonia level >150 μmol/L[12–14]	Neurotoxic effects of plasma ammonia: predicts IH with specificity of 84% and a sensitivity of 60%
3. Plasma ammonia level >200 μmol/L[14]	Neurotoxic effects of plasma ammonia
4. Partial pressure of ammonia or unionized ammonia (pNH3)[12]	Neurotoxic effects of plasma ammonia
5. Sustained elevation on plasma ammonia levels	Neurotoxic effects of plasma ammonia
6. Acute renal failure requiring CRRT[14]	1. Volume overload impeding venous return. 2. Severe acidosis. 3. Decreased clearance of ammonia and glutamine.
7. Young age (<35 y)[14]	Limited intracranial space with limited age related atrophy
8. Vasopressor use[14]	1. Inflammation and multiorgan failure causing vasogenic CE from cerebral hyperemia. 2. Volume overload caused by excessive volume resuscitation.
9. SOFA score[12]	1. Inflammation and multiorgan failure causing vasogenic CE from cerebral hyperemia. 2. Volume overload caused by fluid resuscitation and oliguric renal failure. 3. Decreased ammonia clearance with renal failure. Predicts IH with specificity of 62% and a sensitivity of 94%

CLINICAL AND LABORATORY ASSESSMENT IN OVERT TYPE C HEPATIC ENCEPHALOPATHY (DECOMPENSATED CIRRHOSIS AND ACUTE-ON-CHRONIC LIVER FAILURE)

Precipitating Factors for Overt Type C Hepatic Encephalopathy

Eighty percent of patients with HE have precipitating factors that are reversible. Prompt recognition of precipitating factors and common confounders help identify a reversible cause and refines the approach to investigation and treatment (**Table 5**). Infection was a leading precipitant of episodic and recurrent HE in prior studies and continues to be a major precipitant in ACLF in the recent European Canonic study. This study also found a low incidence of bleeding as a precipitant of HE,[15] which is a paradigm shift from the familiar association of episodic HE with gastrointestinal bleeding in the past.[2] More notably, a distinctive difference in clinical characteristics of patients with HE caused by ACLF versus decompensated cirrhosis was observed (**Table 6**).

Computed Tomography Brain Imaging in Acute Liver Failure and Overt Type B Hepatic Encephalopathy

Utility of brain computed tomography (CT) for assessment of cerebral edema and IH remains unclear, especially when interpretation of CT is performed without a comparator. Imaging is useful for excluding other intracranial processes or evaluating for complications on placing intracranial devices.[16] If imaging is to be used for CE detection

Table 5
Precipitating factors, HE confounders and underlying mechanisms in HE

Mechanism	Precipitating Factor and HE Confounders	Workup to Consider
Excess nitrogen burden	Gastrointestinal bleeding[a] Blood transfusions Constipation[a] Azotemia Excess dietary protein Protein catabolism in starvation and insulin resistance caused by diabetes mellitus[a] Portosystemic shunt[a] (iatrogenic and spontaneous)	Complete blood count blood urea nitrogen and creatinine Micronutrients – B12, B6, thiamine, carnitine level Plasma ammonia levels Blood glucose and HBa1c Abdominal venous imaging
Infection and inflammation	Infection[a] Spontaneous Bacterial Peritonitis[a] Septic shock Viral or autoimmune encephalitis Cryptococcal meningitis Human immunodeficiency virus/AIDS Pancreatitis	Blood, urine, CSF, sputum culture, C difficile toxin Ascitic fluid cell count and culture ScvO2 and lactate Serum and CSF cryptococcus antigen HIV serology Lipase and amylase
Compromised toxin clearance	Dehydration owing to excessive fluid restriction, diuretic use[a], or paracentesis[a], diarrhea Acute kidney injury, hepatorenal syndrome Hypotension owing to bleeding[a] or systemic vasodilatation Abdominal compartment syndrome owing to severe ascites	Renal function Electrolytes (serum sodium) ScvO2 and lactate Monitor bladder pressures
Compromised neurotransmission and metabolism	Endozepines and neurosteroids Benzodiazepine use Coinciding alcohol withdrawal Opioid use Psychoactive drugs Hypoglycemia Hypoxemia and Hypercarbia Thyroid dysfunction	Urine toxicology Blood alcohol level Blood glucose ABG TSH
Acute hepatocellular damage	Alcoholic hepatitis[a] Drugs Other acute hepatitis Development of hepatocellular carcinoma Undiagnosed Wilson's disease	Liver function panel Acetaminophen level Acute hepatitis workup Alpha fetoprotein level Serum and 24-h urinary copper, ceruloplasmin

(continued on next page)

Table 5
(continued)

Mechanism	Precipitating Factor and HE Confounders	Workup to Consider
Other confounders: metabolic abnormalities Neurological injury	IH (subdural hemorrhage is most common cause) Dementia Wernicke's encephalopathy Metronidazole-induced encephalopathy Central pontine myelinolysis Brain stem strokes Severe hyperammonemia Seizure disorder	Head CT Brain MRI with and without gadolinium EEG

Abbreviations: ABG, arterial blood gas; CSF, cerebrospinal fluid; HIV, human immunodeficiency virus; ScvO2, central venous oxygen saturation; TSH, thyroid-stimulating hormone.
  [a] Precipitating factors of HE specific to chronic liver failure.
Data from American Association for the Study of Liver Diseases, European Association for the Study of the Liver. Hepatic encephalopathy in chronic liver disease: 2014 practice guideline by the European Association for the Study of the Liver and the American Association for the Study of Liver Diseases. J Hepatol 2014;61(3):642–59; and Cordoba J, Ventura-Cots M, Simon-Talero M, et al. Characteristics, risk factors, and mortality of cirrhotic patients hospitalized for hepatic encephalopathy with and without acute-on-chronic liver failure (ACLF). J Hepatol 2014;60(2):275–81.

and to assess risk of herniation, performing serial imaging with a baseline scan performed early on before onset of severe HE may be more useful.[17]

Compared with the low prevalence of IH with brain herniation (4%) in ACLF, the increased prevalence of intracranial hemorrhage in ACLF at 23%[9] makes intracranial hemorrhage an important differential to consider. The utility of CT imaging was studied by Joshi and colleagues,[9] who found that among 158 cirrhotic patients scanned for altered mental status, 30% had normal head CT, 30% had increased atrophy, 17% had small vessel disease, and 16% had intracranial hemorrhage.

Table 6
List of Clinical features and precipitating factors for HE in decompensated cirrhosis versus ACLF—Canonic study

	HE in Decompensated Cirrhosis	HE in ACLF
Clinical features	• Older cirrhotics • Inactive drinkers • Less impairment of liver function • Minimal inflammatory reaction • Low prevalence of organ failure • Lower mortality	• Young cirrhotics • More frequently alcoholics • More impairment in liver function • Increased inflammatory response • High prevalence of organ failure • Higher mortality
Precipitating factors	• Long-term diuretic use	• Active alcohol use • Bacterial infections • Hyponatremia

Data from Cordoba J, Ventura-Cots M, Simon-Talero M, et al. Characteristics, risk factors, and mortality of cirrhotic patients hospitalized for hepatic encephalopathy with and without acute-on-chronic liver failure (ACLF). J Hepatol 2014;60(2):275–81.

MRI Brain Imaging in Acute Liver Failure and Overt Type B Hepatic Encephalopathy

Brain MRI may help exclude central nervous system infection, metronidazole encephalopathy, brainstem stoke, Wernicke's encephalopathy, and central pontine myelinolysis not visible on CT and should only be pursued if there is a high index of suspicion. If clinically unstable and MRI is necessary, the patient should be monitored by intensive care unit (ICU) clinicians throughout image acquisition.

A recent MRI finding associated with sustained hyperammonemia reinforces the idea that ammonia is neurotoxic and not just an epiphenomenon in HE.[18,19] Restricted diffusion limited to bilateral insular cortex, cingulate gyrus, and thalamus when mild (limited cortical restricted diffusion [LCRD]) and can involve bilateral temporal, parietal, and frontal lobes and sparing the occipital poles, when severe (diffuse cortical restricted diffusion [DCRD]). This MRI finding is associated with severe hyperammonemia, cognitive decline, matching downstream cortical atrophy, and worse outcome (see **Figs. 1** and **2**).

PHARMACOLOGIC TREATMENT OPTIONS
Invasive Neuromonitoring Strategy in Acute Liver Failure

ICP monitoring has been used to identify and treat elevated ICP aggressively, especially when brain edema was the predominant cause of death.[13,29] With improvement in ICU interventions and lower incidence of IH, the utility of invasive intracranial monitoring has been steadily decreasing. Intracranial hemorrhage from bolt placement is reported to range from 2.5% to 10%.[30,31] Although observational studies have not found overall survival advantages in those receiving ICP monitoring,[32,33] the possibility of benefit in a subset of high-risk brain edema patients remains a possibility. Recombinant factor VII$_a$ is frequently used to help correct the coagulopathy associated with ALF before the procedure.[34,35] When ICP monitoring is performed, the mean cerebral perfusion pressures (CPP) should be maintained between 50 mmHg and 60 mmHg using vasopressors.[25]

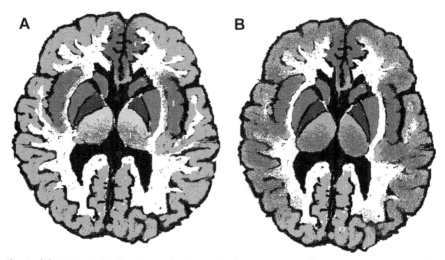

Fig. 1. (A) LCRD—Initial pattern of cytotoxic edema in severe hyperammonemia. Involves insular cortex (I), cingulate gyrus (C), and thalamus (T) with good outcome. (B) DCRD—Diffuse pattern of cytotoxic edema with variable outcome. Involves all cortical grey matter and thalamus with sparing of the occipital poles (O).

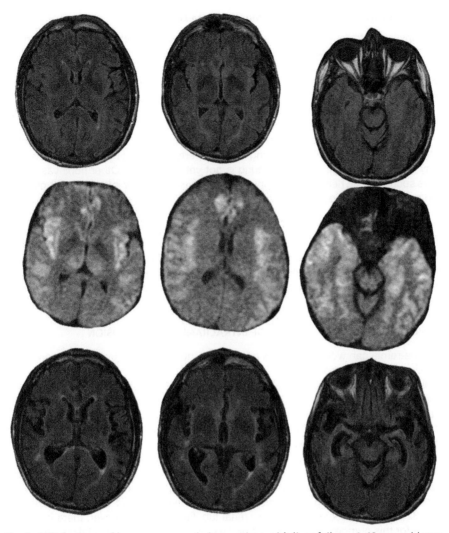

Fig. 2. MRI features of hyperammonemia in a patient with liver failure. A 49-year-old man with hepatitis C, MELD score 17, with accidental chronic acetaminophen overdose, SOFA score 11, and peak plasma NH3 level of 606 μmol/L. Plasma ammonia level was greater than 100 μmol/L for 6 days. (*Top*) Baseline outpatient MRI findings 6 months prior for headache workup. (*Middle*) Diffusion weighted images during admission for liver failure. DCRD involving bilateral cingulate gyrus, insular cortex, temporal lobes, frontal lobes, and posterior thalamus. (*Bottom*) Cortical atrophy matching areas of restricted diffusion on 9-month follow-up MRI. Moderate-to-severe static cognitive impairment. (*From* Kandiah PA, PD, Lynch JR, et al. Catastrophic hyperammonemia: a case series. Neurocritical care 2008;8(1):61–232; and Kandiah PA, Pandya D, Nanchal R, et al. Metaanalysis of magnetic resonance imaging findings and neurological outcomes in liver failure and severe hyperammonemia. In: 15th International Society for Hepatic Encephalopathy and Nitrogen Metabolism: 2012. Grenaa, Denmark, 2012. p. 25–6; with permission.)

Noninvasive Neuromonitoring Strategy in Acute Liver Failure

A noninvasive strategy would be reliant on empiric use of cerebral edema–preventing interventions as listed below without the reassurance of having a pressure reading. Serial CT imaging,[16,36] transcranial Doppler (TCD) ultrasound scan, jugular bulb oximetry, and pupillometry neurological examination are complimentary to this approach.

TCD is a noninvasive method to estimate ICP based on waveform characteristics owing to resistance in cerebral blood flow in proximal cerebral circulation.[37] Its utility in ICP detection in ALF has not been validated prospectively and must be interpreted with caution. Trends in TCD indicating cerebral perfusion could be useful; however, an easy method for continuous monitoring is not yet available.[38] Other noninvasive devices such as optic nerve sonography, technologies using near infrared spectroscopy, and pupillometry have not been validated in ALF.

Neuroprotective Strategies in Acute Liver Failure

Box 1 outlines the approach to preventing and managing cerebral edema in ALF, and **Table 7** delineates organ system considerations that affect cerebrovascular perfusion and development of cerebral edema when treating patients who have ALF. Specific pharmacologic and nonpharmacologic neuroprotective strategies are discussed in the section below.

PREVENTION AND MANAGEMENT OF INTRACRANIAL HYPERTENSION

Hyponatremia can worsen cerebral edema and thus should be treated but care must be taken to avoid rapid correction.

Hypertonic saline used prophylactically to elevate serum sodium level to between 145 and 155 meq/L is found to reduce the incidence and severity of IH in HE grade 3 and 4 patients in a single-center study.[39] Thirty percent hypertonic saline infusion titrated between 5 and 20 mL/h to maintain serum sodium levels at 145 to 155 mmol/L was used in this study.

Hyperosmotic agents have been used traditionally to reduce ICP. This approach may also be used in patients with elevated ICP in ALF patients.[40] Twenty percent mannitol in bolus doses of 0.5 to 1 g/kg body weight can be used to reduce ICP. Serum osmolality should be monitored while on mannitol and should be kept less than 320 mOsm/L because of risk for renal tubular toxicity. However, there is no evidence for this number.[41] Care should be taken in patients with renal failure, as use of mannitol can cause volume overload from osmotic effect of drawing water from the interstitial space.

Hyperventilation causes hypocapnia that induces alkalosis, which, in turn, produces vasoconstriction and thereby a decrease in cerebral blood flow and cerebral blood volume, hence, decreasing ICP. However, there is a serious concern of hypocapnia causing or worsening cerebral ischemia and rebound cerebral edema. Moderate short-term hyperventilation reduces global cerebral blood flow without compromising cerebral oxidative metabolism.[42] Partial pressure of oxygen should be monitored and should be targeted between 30 and 40 mm Hg.[43]

Barbiturate coma may be considered with pentobarbital in selected cases.[44] Thiopental and pentobarbital are found to reduce brain oxygen utilization; however, in the setting of ALF, neurologic assessment cannot be done because of induced coma, and the half-life is prolonged owing to the hepatic metabolism of this drug.

Hypothermia has been successful in decreasing ICP and is reported to help bridge to liver transplant.[45–47] Its use in ALF remains controversial, as 2 studies targeting a

---

Box 1
Outline of management of HE in ALF

I. Identify and treat cause of ALF to minimize further injury

II. Identify risk factors for mortality and IH (see **Table 4**) and evaluate candidacy for liver transplant if high risk

III. Elect neuromonitoring strategy
1. Invasive—intracranial monitoring devices
2. Noninvasive—GCS, neuro checks, pupillary examination, serial brain imaging, TCD, jugular bulb oximetry, optic nerve sonography

IV. Initiate neuroprotective strategies to delay development of CE and IH
1. Head of bed elevation with neck in neutral position
2. Initiate osmotherapy with hypertonic saline or mannitol
   - Crucial to plan an effective osmotherapy strategy taking into account (CRRT)
   - Hypertonic saline with sodium goal of 145 to 150
3. Initiate plasma ammonia–lowering strategies
   - Early initiation of CRRT
   - Targeted temperature management (mild hypothermia 35°C)[20–22]
   - Avoid hypokalemia and metabolic alkalosis[23]
   - Other plasma ammonia–lowering interventions
4. Consider intensive care supportive strategies for multiorgan failure directed at cerebral edema (See Box 1)

V. Rescue maneuvers to control elevated intracranial pressure or refractory IH
1. Maintain adequate cerebral perfusion pressure
   - Vasopressors for shock
2. Increased sedation for metabolic suppression
   - Thiopental or pentobarbital only as a last resort
3. Maximize osmotherapy with hypertonic saline
   - Hypertonic saline with goal sodium of 150 to 155 mmol/L
   - 20% Mannitol with goal osmolality less than 320 mOsm/L
4. Consider continuous neuromuscular blockade infusion for high central venous pressures (>20 mm Hg) or sustained refractory ICP
5. Targeted temperature management (Moderate hypothermia 33–34°C)
6. Consider using indomethacin, 0.5 mg/kg bolus, for refractory ICP
7. Correct severe acidosis with sodium bicarbonate infusions

VI. Slow de-escalation of neuroprotective therapies after liver transplant or in transplant-free recovery
   - IH frequently lag behind liver recovery
   - Slow normalization of serum sodium levels
   - Monitor for rebound edema or dialysis disequilibrium syndrome
   - Slow rewarming to if induced hypothermia initiated

Adapted from Kandiah PA, Olson JC, Subramanian RM. Emerging strategies for treatment of patients with acute hepatic failure. Curr Opin Crit Care 2016;22(2):114; with permission.

---

body temperature of 33–34C, have found both absence of benefit and harm.[22,48] The facilitation of sustained reduction in plasma ammonia levels[46] and slowing the brain metabolism of ammonia and its utility in controlling ICP, remains an attractive intervention in the ICU. Targeting a temperature of 35°C is not an unreasonable approach while reserving lower temperatures for refractory IH or refractory hyperammonemia.

Indomethacin reduced ICP by cerebral vasoconstriction in a porcine model.[49] In a physiologic study of 12 patients with ALF, bolus indomethacin dose of 0.5 mg/kg reduced ICP and increased CPP without compromising cerebral perfusion. Further studies need to be performed before considering it for routine use.

Table 7
Intensive care supportive strategies directed at cerebral edema in ALF

Organ System	Intensive Care Supportive Strategies
Neurologic	Use short-acting sedatives and opiates once intubated. Propofol and low-dose fentanyl are sedatives of choice. Avoid intermediate or long-acting benzodiazepines.
Respiratory	Intubation for airway protection needs to be considered early in later stages of HE before significant aspiration and lung injury occurs. Low tidal volume lung protective strategy to prevent ARDS. High intrathoracic pressures result in cerebral venous outflow obstruction.[24] High PEEP → use cautiously as very high PEEP can theoretically add to hepatic congestion. PEEP <15 has not been shown to affect ICP significantly. CO_2 goal: 30–40 mm Hg → hypercarbia causes vasodilatation
Cardiovascular	Noninvasive approach and IH suspected → target a higher MAP goal ($\geq$80 mm Hg) Invasive approach → CPP should be maintained between 50 and 60 using vasopressors.[25] In refractory shock → consider plasma exchange to maintain optimal CPP. Plasma exchange was associated with reduction in SIRS response, reduction in SOFA scores and decline in need for vasopressor support.[21,26] CVP goal <20 → increased CVP may impede venous return from the brain.[27] Maintain euvolemia. Consider paralysis.
Renal, acid base disorders and electrolytes	Early CRRT → to maintain euvolemia, augment ammonia clearance,[28] correction of electrolyte and acidosis correction. Formulate strategy to maintain sodium goal (145–150) while on CRRT. Options include preparation of hypertonic PrismaSate or hypertonic saline infusion in postfilter return arm of CRRT. Caution: Initiating CRRT with isotonic PrismaSate in patient with IH and induced hypernatremia can cause rebound edema from dialysis disequilibrium syndrome and precipitate brain herniation. Hypokalemia and metabolic acidosis increase renal ammonia production. Metabolic alkalosis promotes formation of NH_3 from (NH_4^+) augmenting its passage across the blood-brain barrier.[14,15]
Gastrointestinal, liver, and nutrition	Abdominal compartment syndrome may indirectly worsen ICP. Lactulose → avoid lactulose via oral or nasogastric route in ALF, as it may cause bowel distention, worsening ileus, and complicating transplant surgery. Limited evidence supporting it use in ALF. If used, it is safer to be given rectally.
Endocrine	Avoid hypoglycemia → may add to metabolic injury to the brain. Initiate 10% dextrose or 20% dextrose pre-emptively in ALF.
Hematologic and immune system	DIC → consider repeating head CT if DIC occurs, as spontaneous intracranial hemorrhages may occur.

Abbreviations: ARDS, acute respiratory distress syndrome; CVP, central venous pressure; DIC, disseminated intravascular coagulation; MAP, mean arterial pressure; PEEP, positive end-expiratory pressure; SIRS, systemic inflammatory response syndrome.

Seizures can worsen cerebral edema and increase ICP. Because one-third of patients with ALF has seizures, continuous electroencephalogram (EEG) monitoring should be considered in patients who are both sedated and paralyzed.[50] Phenytoin was found to reduce breakthrough seizures in one small study, whereas using it prophylactically was of no benefit in another.[51] Although phenytoin is indicated in breakthrough seizures in ALF, it is not unreasonable to consider the use of newer anti-epileptic medications with fewer side-effect profiles and not metabolized by the liver.

Continuous reno-renal replacement therapy (CRRT) is recommended over hemodialysis because of lower fluctuations in ICP and improved hemodynamic stability. CRRT is particularly effective at lowering plasma ammonia levels[28] and correcting hyponatremia. Appropriate consideration should be given to sodium concentration in Prismasate with dialysate for CRRT and intravenous hypertonic saline dosing when determining desired serum sodium level.

PLASMA AMMONIA–LOWERING STRATEGIES IN ACUTE LIVER FAILURE

Ammonia plays a significant but fragmented role in the development of cerebral edema and IH. There remains a paucity of studies that show therapeutic benefit to ammonia reduction. Although drugs given for chronic HE, including lactulose and rifaximin, may offer a nominal plasma ammonia reduction effect, they are likely deficient in preventing IH in ALF. Unlike cirrhosis, ALF patients are not preconditioned to deal with hyperammonemia and are likely more susceptible to ammonia-related toxicity. In practice, plasma ammonia reduction in ALF has been orchestrated habitually and serendipitously by using CRRT[28] and therapeutic hypothermia.[46]

THERAPEUTIC STRATEGIES FOR MANAGING TYPE C HEPATIC ENCEPHALOPATHY IN THE INTENSIVE CARE UNIT

Box 2 outlines the approach to managing HE in chronic liver failure. Specific pharmacologic and nonpharmacologic therapies for management of HE include the following.

Plasma Ammonia–Lowering Strategies

Reduction of intestinal ammonia production and absorption
Lactulose (β-galactofructose) and lactitol (β-galactosidosorbitol) Despite the absence of mortality benefit, both these nonabsorbable disaccharides are currently first-line agents for the treatment of HE. Lactitol is not available in the United States. Lactulose is superior to placebo and tap water enemas and comparable to neomycin.[52,53] Lactulose favors conversion of NH_3 to NH_4^+, which is relatively membrane impermeable and less absorbed, inhibits ammoniagenic coliform bacteria by acidifying the gut, and clears ammonia by decreasing transit time.

Box 2
Goals of therapy for HE in chronic liver failure

I. Identification of HE presenting with decompensated cirrhosis versus ACLF
   1. ACLF patient will require earlier transfer to the ICU because of imminent mortality

II. Treatment of precipitating factors in parallel with intensive care supportive strategies for multiorgan failure

III. Initiation of first-tier therapeutic strategies specific to HE
   1. Reduction of intestinal ammonia production and absorption
   2. Nutritional and micronutrient supplementation

IV. Initiation of second-tier therapeutic strategies specific to HE
   1. Plasma ammonia–lowering devices and nonpharmacologic interventions
   2. Eliminating large spontaneous portosystemic shunts
      • Ideal for low MELD score candidates
   3. Alternative pathway therapies
   4. Neurotransmitter blockade

Dosage is oral or via nasogastric tube, 45 mL initially followed by repeated dose every hour until the patient has a bowel movement. The treatment is more appropriate in patients who are alert or intubated with low aspiration risk. Once bowel movement achieved, lactulose is titrated (15–45 mL every 8–12 hours) to achieve 3 soft bowel movements per day. Production of liquid stool should be avoided, as it will worsen the patients' nutritional status and promote further catabolism.

A 300-mL enema in 700 mL water retained for 1 hour in Trendelenburg position is done. This treatment is more appropriate in patients with grade 3 to 4 encephalopathy in which risk of aspiration is high.

Polyethylene glycol A small, randomized single-center study found that 4 L of *polyethylene* glycol administered orally or nasogastrically over 4 hours led to more rapid HE resolution despite less ammonia difference at 24 hours compared with standard therapy with lactulose.[54] Polyethylene glycol's safety profile and balanced electrolytes make it an attractive adjunct to lactulose in the ICU setting. A volume of 4 L remains a concern for aspiration, especially in later grades of HE.

Ammonia-lowering antibiotics

Rifaximin Rifaximin is US Food and Drug Administration (FDA) approved for HE prevention in compensated cirrhosis. Rifaximin is an oral nonsystemic antibiotic with less than 0.4% absorption. Although there is strong evidence supporting the use of rifaximin as secondary prophylactically for overt HE in compensated cirrhosis,[55] its use in overt HE is contentious. Numerous small studies have attempted to validate the use of rifaximin in overt HE. Lactulose and rifaximin was found to be equally effective at preventing HE when used prophylactically in acute variceal bleeding.[56] In treating type B HE grade I to III, rifaximin was as effective as lactitol, with both achieving an efficacy of greater than 80%.[57] Rifaximin was also more efficacious in reducing plasma ammonia levels and improving EEG findings. The largest of these randomized, controlled trials was by Sharma and colleagues (n = 120) comparing rifaximin and lactulose with lactulose and placebo in which 80% of patients had severe HE.[58] A higher proportion of complete HE reversal, shorter hospital stays, and improvement in 10-day mortality rate was reported. In the absence of more robust multicenter studies, rifaximin (550 mg orally twice per day) is a reasonable adjunct for severe or refractory HE and has a better side-effect profile compared with neomycin and metronidazole.

Neomycin Neomycin is FDA approved for the management of acute HE despite small and conflicting studies supporting its use.[59,60] The dosage is 1000 mg every 6 hours for up to 6 days in acute HE; 1–2 g daily for chronic HE may be used. Despite its poor absorption, chronic administration can result in nephrotoxicity and ototoxicity.

Metronidazole Metronidazole is not FDA approved for management of HE. One small study found that it is as effective as neomycin at a dose of 250 mg twice daily.[61] The concerns for resistant *Clostridium difficile* colitis and neurotoxic effects of metronidazole are valid.

Plasma ammonia–lowering devices and nonpharmacologic interventions

Continuous renal replacement therapy Continuous renal replacement therapy using continuous veno-venous hemofiltration with high filtration volume (90 mL/kg/h) is an effective method of rapidly lowering serum plasma ammonia levels.[28,62] Ammonia clearance is closely associated with ultrafiltration rate. Instituting CRRT for acute renal failure is perfectly acceptable; however, initiating it predominantly for refractory hyperammonemia in cirrhosis is a practice not supported by any clinical study. If approached from the paradigm of a toxidrome, a case can be made for it. How would one approach a dialyzable toxin, refractory to medications, if at extreme levels can cause irreversible brain injury, persistent coma, and, in rare instances, IH with transtentorial herniation?

Molecular adsorbent recirculating system Molecular adsorbent recirculating system is a blood detoxification system based on albumin dialysis that removes protein bound (bile acids, bilirubin, endozepines, nitrous oxide) and water soluble toxins (ammonia, creatinine). In the United States, MARS is FDA approved for management of ALF caused by drug overdose or toxic exposures and for management of HE in decompensated cirrhosis. MARS trials thus far have failed to show a survival benefit; however, 3 main trials have consistently found improvement in HE and a satisfactory safety profile. Using MARS for refractory HE is a reasonable and safe option.

Therapeutic hypothermia (goal temperature of 34°C) There remains limited clinical experience in the use of mild hypothermia in chronic liver failure.[63] Its appeal in liver disease is that it counteracts many of the metabolic effects of ammonia and slows protein catabolism and production of ammonia by bacteria and the kidneys.[64,65] The predominant concern with using hypothermia in cirrhotic patients is its potential to worsen the existing coagulopathy in patients who are at high risk for variceal bleeding and the predisposition to infection. In rare cases of extreme refractory hyperammonemia, hypothermia could be used as a transient neuroprotective strategy while pursuing clearance of plasma ammonia through other avenues.

Embolizing large spontaneous portosystemic shunts
Two retrospective series found safety and efficacy of embolization in large portosystemic shunts in refractory HE. Fifty-nine percent (n = 37) were free from HE within 100 days, and 48% were free from HE for more than 2 years. In the second study, 90% (n = 15) improved 2 months after the procedure. Median Model for End-Stage Liver disease (MELD) score in both studies was 13. MELD score of more than 11 was associated with increased risk recurrence of HE.

Alternative pathway therapy
Multiple ongoing studies are evaluating the utility of ornithine phenylacetate, which shows some promise. There are insufficient robust studies looking at utility of L-ornithine L-aspartate in overt HE. One south Asian study using L-ornithine L-aspartate as adjunctive therapy in patients with HE grade II found improvement in grade of HE.

Neurotransmitter blockade
In a systematic review involving 13 controlled trials with a total of 805 patients, the use of flumazenil was associated with significant improvement in HE but failed to show long-term benefits or improvement in outcome.[66] As a short-acting benzodiazepine antagonist, flumazenil is postulated to inhibit endogenous GABAergic substances and previous residual effects of long-acting benzodiazepine. Cirrhotics are also found to have increased benzodiazepine receptor activation, but only a subset of patients will show response to flumazenil. Flumazenil should be used in a closely monitored environment, as it has a potential of provoking seizures.

A trial of 1–2 mg of flumazenil in 20-mL saline solution by intravenous infusion for 3 to 5 minutes may be considered in patients with stage 3 to 4 encephalopathy who have low serum ammonia level and have not responded to lactulose.

Nutritional and micronutrient supplementation
There are numerous anecdotal reports and small studies about the ammonia-lowering effects of oral supplementation with zinc and carnitine, which require further study.

SURGICAL TREATMENT OPTIONS

Liver transplantation is the definitive treatment for HE.[67] It is important to differentiate between those patients who will recover spontaneously and those who will not. The 1-year survival rates after liver transplant are greater than 80% in United States.

SUMMARY

Transplantation aside, mortality reduction in subsets of liver failure are not attributable to any single therapeutic intervention but is perhaps the net result of many critical care interventions. Modest benefits from newer therapies may collectively continue to improve outcomes in acute and chronic liver failure.

REFERENCES

1. Ferenci P, Lockwood A, Mullen K, et al. Hepatic encephalopathy–definition, nomenclature, diagnosis, and quantification: final report of the working party at the 11th World Congresses of Gastroenterology, Vienna, 1998. Hepatology 2002;35(3):716–21.

2. American Association for the Study of Liver Diseases, European Association for the Study of the Liver. Hepatic encephalopathy in chronic liver disease: 2014 practice guideline by the European Association for the Study of the Liver and the American Association for the Study of Liver Diseases. J Hepatol 2014; 61(3):642–59.

3. O'Grady J. Modern management of acute liver failure. Clin Liver Dis 2007;11(2): 291–303.

4. Bernal W, Hyyrylainen A, Gera A, et al. Lessons from look-back in acute liver failure? A single centre experience of 3300 patients. J Hepatol 2013;59(1):74–80.

5. Romero-Gomez M, Montagnese S, Jalan R. Hepatic encephalopathy in patients with acute decompensation of cirrhosis and acute-on-chronic liver failure. J Hepatol 2015;62(2):437–47.

6. Donovan JP, Schafer DF, Shaw BW Jr, et al. Cerebral oedema and increased intracranial pressure in chronic liver disease. Lancet 1998;351(9104):719–21.

7. Jalan R, Bernuau J. Induction of cerebral hyperemia by ammonia plus endotoxin: does hyperammonemia unlock the blood-brain barrier? J Hepatol 2007;47(2): 168–71.

8. Jalan R, Dabos K, Redhead DN, et al. Elevation of intracranial pressure following transjugular intrahepatic portosystemic stent-shunt for variceal haemorrhage. J Hepatol 1997;27(5):928–33.

9. Joshi D, O'Grady J, Patel A, et al. Cerebral oedema is rare in acute-on-chronic liver failure patients presenting with high-grade hepatic encephalopathy. Liver Int 2014;34(3):362–6.

10. Conn HBJ. Quantifying the severity of Hepatic encephalopathy. Bloomington (IL): Medi-Ed Press; 1994.

11. Yan S, Tu Z, Lu W, et al. Clinical utility of an automated pupillometer for assessing and monitoring recipients of liver transplantation. Liver Transpl 2009;15(12): 1718–27.

12. Kitzberger R, Funk GC, Holzinger U, et al. Severity of organ failure is an independent predictor of intracranial hypertension in acute liver failure. Clin Gastroenterol Hepatol 2009;7(9):1000–6.

13. Clemmesen JO, Larsen FS, Kondrup J, et al. Cerebral herniation in patients with acute liver failure is correlated with arterial ammonia concentration. Hepatology 1999;29(3):648–53.
14. Bernal W, Hall C, Karvellas CJ, et al. Arterial ammonia and clinical risk factors for encephalopathy and intracranial hypertension in acute liver failure. Hepatology 2007;46(6):1844–52.
15. Cordoba J, Ventura-Cots M, Simon-Talero M, et al. Characteristics, risk factors, and mortality of cirrhotic patients hospitalized for hepatic encephalopathy with and without acute-on-chronic liver failure (ACLF). J Hepatol 2014;60(2):275–81.
16. Munoz SJ, Robinson M, Northrup B, et al. Elevated intracranial pressure and computed tomography of the brain in fulminant hepatocellular failure. Hepatology 1991;13(2):209–12.
17. Thayapararajah SW, Gulka I, Al-Amri A, et al. Acute fulminant hepatic failure, encephalopathy and early CT changes. Can J Neurol Sci 2013;40(4):553–7.
18. McKinney AM, Lohman BD, Sarikaya B, et al. Acute hepatic encephalopathy, diffusion-weighted and fluid-attenuated inversion recovery findings, and correlation with plasma ammonia level and clinical outcome. AJNR Am J Neuroradiol 2010;31(8):1471–9.
19. U-King-Im JM, Yu E, Bartlett E, et al. Acute hyperammonemic encephalopathy in adults: imaging findings. AJNR Am J Neuroradiol 2011;32(2):413–8.
20. Bernal W, Wendon J. Acute liver failure. N Engl J Med 2014;370(12):1170–1.
21. Larsen FS, Schmidt LE, Bernsmeier C, et al. High-volume plasma exchange in patients with acute liver failure: an open randomised controlled trial. J Hepatol 2015;64(1):69–78.
22. Karvellas CJ, Todd Stravitz R, Battenhouse H, et al. Therapeutic hypothermia in acute liver failure: a multicenter retrospective cohort analysis. Liver Transpl 2015;21(1):4–12.
23. Tapper EB, Jiang ZG, Patwardhan VR. Refining the ammonia hypothesis: a physiology-driven approach to the treatment of hepatic encephalopathy. Mayo Clin Proc 2015;90(5):646–58.
24. Citerio G, Vascotto E, Villa F, et al. Induced abdominal compartment syndrome increases intracranial pressure in neurotrauma patients: a prospective study. Crit Care Med 2001;29(7):1466–71.
25. Polson J, Lee WM, American Association for the Study of Liver Disease. AASLD position paper: the management of acute liver failure. Hepatology 2005;41(5):1179–97.
26. Larsen FS, Hansen BA, Ejlersen E, et al. Cerebral blood flow, oxygen metabolism and transcranial Doppler sonography during high-volume plasmapheresis in fulminant hepatic failure. Eur J Gastroenterol Hepatol 1996;8(3):261–5.
27. Scheuermann K, Thiel C, Thiel K, et al. Correlation of the intracranial pressure to the central venous pressure in the late phase of acute liver failure in a porcine model. Acta Neurochir Suppl 2012;114:387–91.
28. Slack AJ, Auzinger G, Willars C, et al. Ammonia clearance with haemofiltration in adults with liver disease. Liver Int 2014;34(1):42–8.
29. Keays RT, Alexander GJ, Williams R. The safety and value of extradural intracranial pressure monitors in fulminant hepatic failure. J Hepatol 1993;18(2):205–9.
30. Vaquero J, Fontana RJ, Larson AM, et al. Complications and use of intracranial pressure monitoring in patients with acute liver failure and severe encephalopathy. Liver Transpl 2005;11(12):1581–9.
31. Blei AT, Olafsson S, Webster S, et al. Complications of intracranial pressure monitoring in fulminant hepatic failure. Lancet 1993;341(8838):157–8.

32. Lidofsky SD, Bass NM, Prager MC, et al. Intracranial pressure monitoring and liver transplantation for fulminant hepatic failure. Hepatology 1992;16(1):1–7.

33. Karvellas CJ, Fix OK, Battenhouse H, et al, US Acute Liver Failure Study Group. Outcomes and complications of intracranial pressure monitoring in acute liver failure: a retrospective cohort study. Crit Care Med 2014;42(5):1157–67.

34. Kositchaiwat C, Chuansumrit A. Experiences with recombinant factor VIIa for the prevention of bleeding in patients with chronic liver disease undergoing percutaneous liver biopsies and endoscopic retrograde cholangiopancreatography (ERCP). Thromb Haemost 2001;86(4):1125–6.

35. Shami VM, Caldwell SH, Hespenheide EE, et al. Recombinant activated factor VII for coagulopathy in fulminant hepatic failure compared with conventional therapy. Liver Transpl 2003;9(2):138–43.

36. Wijdicks EF, Plevak DJ, Rakela J, et al. Clinical and radiologic features of cerebral edema in fulminant hepatic failure. Mayo Clin Proc 1995;70(2):119–24.

37. Aggarwal S, Brooks DM, Kang Y, et al. Noninvasive monitoring of cerebral perfusion pressure in patients with acute liver failure using transcranial doppler ultrasonography. Liver Transpl 2008;14(7):1048–57.

38. Abdo A, Lopez O, Fernandez A, et al. Transcranial Doppler sonography in fulminant hepatic failure. Transplant Proc 2003;35(5):1859–60.

39. Murphy N, Auzinger G, Bernel W, et al. The effect of hypertonic sodium chloride on intracranial pressure in patients with acute liver failure. Hepatology 2004; 39(2):464–70.

40. Canalese J, Gimson AE, Davis C, et al. Controlled trial of dexamethasone and mannitol for the cerebral oedema of fulminant hepatic failure. Gut 1982;23(7): 625–9.

41. Diringer MN, Zazulia AR. Osmotic therapy: fact and fiction. Neurocrit Care 2004; 1(2):219–33.

42. Strauss GI. The effect of hyperventilation upon cerebral blood flow and metabolism in patients with fulminant hepatic failure. Dan Med Bull 2007;54(2):99–111.

43. Ede RJ, Gimson AE, Bihari D, et al. Controlled hyperventilation in the prevention of cerebral oedema in fulminant hepatic failure. J Hepatol 1986;2(1):43–51.

44. Forbes A, Alexander GJ, O'Grady JG, et al. Thiopental infusion in the treatment of intracranial hypertension complicating fulminant hepatic failure. Hepatology 1989;10(3):306–10.

45. Jalan R, O Damink SW, Deutz NE, et al. Moderate hypothermia for uncontrolled intracranial hypertension in acute liver failure. Lancet 1999;354(9185):1164–8.

46. Jalan R, Olde Damink SW, Deutz NE, et al. Moderate hypothermia in patients with acute liver failure and uncontrolled intracranial hypertension. Gastroenterology 2004;127(5):1338–46.

47. Vaquero J. Therapeutic hypothermia in the management of acute liver failure. Neurochem Int 2012;60(7):723–35.

48. Larsen FS, MN, Bernal W, et al; EUROALF Group. The prophylactive effect of mild hypothermia to prevent brain edema in patients with acute liver failure: results of a multicenter randomized, controlled trial [abstract]. J Hepatol 54(Suppl 1):S26.

49. Tofteng F, Larsen FS. The effect of indomethacin on intracranial pressure, cerebral perfusion and extracellular lactate and glutamate concentrations in patients with fulminant hepatic failure. J Cereb Blood Flow Metab 2004;24(7):798–804.

50. Ellis AJ, Wendon JA, Williams R. Subclinical seizure activity and prophylactic phenytoin infusion in acute liver failure: a controlled clinical trial. Hepatology 2000;32(3):536–41.

51. Bhatia V, Batra Y, Acharya SK. Prophylactic phenytoin does not improve cerebral edema or survival in acute liver failure–a controlled clinical trial. J Hepatol 2004; 41(1):89–96.
52. Als-Nielsen B, Gluud LL, Gluud C. Nonabsorbable disaccharides for hepatic encephalopathy. Cochrane Database Syst Rev 2004;(2):CD003044.
53. Uribe M, Campollo O, Vargas F, et al. Acidifying enemas (lactitol and lactose) vs. nonacidifying enemas (tap water) to treat acute portal-systemic encephalopathy: a double-blind, randomized clinical trial. Hepatology 1987;7(4):639–43.
54. Rahimi RS, Cuthbert JA, Rockey DC. Lactulose vs polyethylene glycol for treatment of hepatic encephalopathy-reply. JAMA Intern Med 2015;175(5):868–9.
55. Bass NM, Mullen KD, Sanyal A, et al. Rifaximin treatment in hepatic encephalopathy. N Engl J Med 2010;362(12):1071–81.
56. Maharshi S, Sharma BC, Srivastava S, et al. Randomised controlled trial of lactulose versus rifaximin for prophylaxis of hepatic encephalopathy in patients with acute variceal bleed. Gut 2015;64(8):1341–2.
57. Mas A, Rodes J, Sunyer L, et al. Comparison of rifaximin and lactitol in the treatment of acute hepatic encephalopathy: results of a randomized, double-blind, double-dummy, controlled clinical trial. J Hepatol 2003;38(1):51–8.
58. Conn HO, Leevy CM, Vlahcevic ZR, et al. Comparison of lactulose and neomycin in the treatment of chronic portal-systemic encephalopathy. A double blind controlled trial. Gastroenterology 1977;72(4 Pt 1):573–83.
59. Sharma BC, Sharma P, Lunia MK, et al. A randomized, double-blind, controlled trial comparing rifaximin plus lactulose with lactulose alone in treatment of overt hepatic encephalopathy. Am J Gastroenterol 2013;108(9):1458–63.
60. Strauss E, Tramote R, Silva EP, et al. Double-blind randomized clinical trial comparing neomycin and placebo in the treatment of exogenous hepatic encephalopathy. Hepatogastroenterology 1992;39(6):542–5.
61. Morgan MH, Read AE, Speller DC. Treatment of hepatic encephalopathy with metronidazole. Gut 1982;23(1):1–7.
62. Cordoba J, Blei AT, Mujais S. Determinants of ammonia clearance by hemodialysis. Artif Organs 1996;20(7):800–3.
63. Chawla R, Smith D, Marik PE. Near fatal posterior reversible encephalopathy syndrome complicating chronic liver failure and treated by induced hypothermia and dialysis: a case report. J Med Case Rep 2009;3:6623.
64. Vaquero J, Butterworth RF. Mechanisms of brain edema in acute liver failure and impact of novel therapeutic interventions. Neurol Res 2007;29(7):683–90.
65. Vaquero J, Blei AT. Mild hypothermia for acute liver failure: a review of mechanisms of action. J Clin Gastroenterol 2005;39(4 Suppl 2):S147–57.
66. Als-Nielsen B, Gluud LL, Gluud C. Benzodiazepine receptor antagonists for hepatic encephalopathy. Cochrane Database Syst Rev 2004;(2):CD002798.
67. Keays R, Potter D, O'Grady J, et al. Intracranial and cerebral perfusion pressure changes before, during and immediately after orthotopic liver transplantation for fulminant hepatic failure. Q J Med 1991;79(289):425–33.

The Circulatory System in Liver Disease

Steven M. Hollenberg, MD*, Brett Waldman, MD

KEYWORDS

- Circulation • Liver disease • Cirrhosis • Vascular resistance

KEY POINTS

- Liver failure is a hyperdynamic state, characterized by a decrease in systemic vascular resistance and increase in cardiac output and heart rate.
- This hyperdynamic state results from splanchnic arterial vasodilatation and opening of portosystemic collaterals, which is mostly mediated by overproduction of nitric oxide and other vasoactive substances.
- Cardiac cirrhosis (congestive hepatopathy) is liver dysfunction consequent to right-sided heart failure.
- Despite a hyperdynamic state, latent cardiac dysfunction, termed cirrhotic cardiomyopathy, may develop and may be manifested by decreased cardiac reserve.
- Latent cardiomyopathy may cause heart failure or hemodynamic decompensation in conditions of stress such as infection, postoperatively, or after transjugular intrahepatic portosystemic shunt placement. Cirrhotic cardiomyopathy may be reversible following liver transplant.

In the cirrhotic liver, distortion of the normal liver architecture occurs as a result of both structural and vascular changes. Because of the arterial vasodilatation that occurs mainly in the systemic and splanchnic circulation, portal hypertension is often associated with a hyperdynamic circulatory syndrome in which cardiac output (CO) and heart rate are increased and systemic vascular resistance (SVR) is decreased. The release of several vasoactive substances, most notably nitric oxide (NO), is considered to be the primary factor involved in the reduction of mesenteric arterial resistance. This decrease in effective circulatory volume triggers baroreceptor-mediated activation of the sympathetic nervous system (SNS) and renin-angiotensin-aldosterone system (RAAS), resulting in sodium and water retention with eventual formation of ascites. The hyperdynamic circulatory state also contributes to numerous cardiovascular abnormalities, including diastolic dysfunction, blunted systolic response to stress, and electrophysiologic abnormalities, which together have been termed cirrhotic cardiomyopathy.

Department of Cardiovascular Disease, Cooper University Hospital, 1 Cooper Plaza, Camden, 08103, NJ, USA
* Corresponding author.
E-mail address: hollenberg-steven@cooperhealth.edu

Crit Care Clin 32 (2016) 331–342
http://dx.doi.org/10.1016/j.ccc.2016.02.004
0749-0704/16/$ – see front matter
criticalcare.theclinics.com

Echocardiography is a useful imaging modality for evaluation of latent cardiac disease in cirrhotic patients as well as for assessment of comorbidities such as pulmonary hypertension and hepatopulmonary syndrome. The clinical manifestations of cirrhotic cardiomyopathy may become apparent during certain procedures and surgeries, as well as infection, when added stress is placed on the cardiovascular system. Management of these patients with acute cardiac dysfunction can be challenging and often requires invasive hemodynamic monitoring in an intensive care unit (ICU) setting to tailor decisions regarding use of fluids and vasopressors.

PATHOPHYSIOLOGY OF PORTAL HYPERTENSION

The liver normally has high compliance and low resistance that accommodates large volumes of blood, as may occur after eating, without a significant increase in portal pressure. Portal hypertension develops as a result of increases in both portal resistance and portal inflow. Cirrhosis increases resistance to portal flow as a result of collagen deposition in the hepatic acinus, which markedly reduces the total cross-sectional area of the hepatic sinusoids by narrowing the sinusoidal lumen.[1] Intrahepatic portal resistance is further increased by compression of the central veins by portal inflammation and regenerating nodules. This increase in resistance to portal outflow leads to the opening of a portosystemic collateral circulation that occurs through dilatation of preexisting vessels and also by angiogenesis in an attempt to reduce portal pressures. Ultimately, these portosystemic shunts are insufficient at normalizing portal pressures, and complications of portal hypertension, such as gastroesophageal varices and hepatic encephalopathy, can ensue.[1,2]

HYPERDYNAMIC CIRCULATORY SYNDROME

Liver failure is a hyperdynamic state, with increased CO, decreased SVR, and normal or decreased blood pressure (**Box 1**). The chief cause of the hyperdynamic circulation is vasodilatation, which occurs in both the systemic and splanchnic circulations. The consequent reduction in SVR leads to an increase in CO, and blood pressure can be reduced as well. Although extracellular fluid volume is increased, circulating blood volume is decreased. In order to maintain hemodynamic homeostasis, CO and heart rate are increased.

Portal hypertension plays a pivotal role in the development of hyperdynamic circulatory syndrome in patients with advanced liver disease. The increased resistance to portal inflow and outflow contributes to systemic and splanchnic vasodilatation. Portal hypertension may also allow intestinal vasoactive substances to bypass the liver and reach the systemic circulation.

According to the peripheral arterial vasodilatation hypothesis, the decrease in SVR that occurs is a result of peripheral vasodilatation that triggers activation of

---

Box 1
Hyperdynamic circulatory syndrome

- Increased plasma volume
- Increased CO
- Increased heart rate
- Decreased SVR
- Normal or decreased mean arterial blood pressure

compensatory neurohormonal pathways, including the RAAS and SNS, leading to salt and water retention. As a result, the total blood volume is increased but abnormally distributed throughout the vasculature, leading to a decreased effective blood volume. Specifically, the central arterial blood volume supplying the heart and lungs is decreased and noncentral blood volume in the splanchnic circulation is increased.[3] In a study in which cirrhotic patients received volume expansion by intravenous infusion of hyperosmotic galactose, central blood volume increased in patients with mild cirrhosis. In contrast, in patients with advanced cirrhosis (Child-Turcotte class B and C), central blood volume did not expand in response to volume load despite increases in CO and noncentral blood volume.[4] These findings suggest that volume expansion by itself does not account for the increase in CO seen in cirrhotic patients. The abnormal distribution of blood volume in cirrhosis is likely caused by imbalances of endogenous vasoconstrictors (such as norepinephrine, vasopressin) and vasodilators (such as NO) in various vascular beds.[4] Thus, a decrease in effective arterial volume combined with increased venous return to the heart through portosystemic shunts maintains a high CO state.[5] As liver disease and vasodilatation worsen, the heart may be unable to compensate, especially during stress, resulting in cardiac dysfunction.

Collateral Circulation

The formation of portosystemic shunts also plays a major role in the development of hyperdynamic circulation by reducing peripheral resistance and allowing direct passage of vasoactive substances into the systemic circulation.[1] This collateral circulation develops in response to the increase in portal pressures that occurs in cirrhotic patients. As portal pressures exceed the systemic venous pressure, flow in these collateral vessels is reversed and blood flows out of the portal circulation toward the systemic venous circulation. Angiogenic factors such as vascular endothelial growth factor (VEGF) also have a role in formation of collaterals. Increased flow through these collaterals occurs as a result of splanchnic vasodilatation and increased portal blood inflow, leading to variceal expansion and eventual rupture.[6] Although portosystemic collaterals develop at various sites throughout the body (ie, umbilicus and rectum), the most clinically relevant are gastroesophageal varices, which are present in almost half of patients with cirrhosis at the time of diagnosis. Variceal hemorrhage is the most lethal complication of cirrhosis.

Proposed Mechanisms for Splanchnic Vasodilatation

Several vasoactive substances and systems have been extensively investigated as potential mediators of splanchnic vasodilatation. In particular, NO plays a critical role in the reduction of mesenteric and systemic arterial resistance, which leads to the hyperdynamic circulatory syndrome in cirrhosis.[1] Some studies have suggested that serum nitrate levels can be used to predict progression of liver failure because higher levels of nitrate correlate with more advanced stages of cirrhosis.[7,8] NO diffuses freely across cell membranes and triggers relaxation of smooth muscle cells via stimulation of guanylate cyclase with subsequent increase in cyclic GMP. There are several proposed mechanisms for the increased production of NO in the splanchnic circulation of cirrhotic patients[1,2]:

- Increased shear stress in the mesenteric circulation caused by portal hypertension may indirectly increase NO synthase (NOS) activity through various signaling cascades.
- Bacterial translocation from the gut into mesenteric lymph nodes in patients with cirrhosis may increase NO production.

- Inflammatory cytokines and VEGF activation of NOS.[1,9]

In addition to NO, numerous other molecules have been shown to participate in vasodilatation, including carbon monoxide, prostacyclin, and endocannabinoids (see **Fig. 2**).

FLUID RETENTION IN LIVER FAILURE

The development of ascites is the most common complication of end-stage liver disease and is associated with significant mortality; 1-year and 5-year survivals are 85% and 56%, respectively.[10,11] The peripheral arterial vasodilatation theory is the most widely accepted explanation for the formation of ascites in cirrhosis. Portal hypertension triggers splanchnic and peripheral arterial vasodilatation, mostly mediated by NO overproduction. This arterial vasodilatation leads to effective underfilling of the systemic vascular space, resulting in a decrease in arterial blood pressure. In contrast, vascular resistance may be normal or increased in other vascular beds (ie, kidney, brain, muscles), depending on the degree of liver impairment. In an effort to restore normal circulatory flow, baroreceptor-mediated activation of the RAAS, aldosterone, and SNS occurs, leading to avid sodium and water retention (**Fig. 1**). As liver disease worsens, fluid accumulates in the form of edema, pleural effusions, and ascites.

Determining the Cause of Ascites

Although cirrhosis accounts for more than 75% of patients presenting with ascites, the remaining 25% of cases are caused by malignancy, heart failure, tuberculosis, and other rare causes,[12,13] and so diagnostic paracentesis should be done in patients with new-onset ascites and sent for quantification of protein and albumin concentrations, cell count, culture, and cytology. Calculation of the serum-ascites albumin gradient (SAAG; the serum albumin concentration relative to the albumin concentration in ascitic fluid) can help distinguish ascites related to portal (sinusoidal) hypertension from all other causes of ascitic fluid collection, such as malignancy. The SAAG value is a measurement of the balance of oncotic forces that exist between the vascular space and peritoneal space. Normally, serum oncotic pressure is in equilibrium with serum hydrostatic pressure. In portal hypertension, increased hydrostatic pressure causes fluid to move from the circulation into the peritoneal space, concentrating the serum albumin and thus increasing the SAAG value. The SAAG calculation has been proved to be superior to the older total protein–based method of categorizing ascitic fluid as transudative or exudative based on ascitic protein concentration (<2.5 g/dL or >2.5 g/dL).[14,15]

Cardiac Dysfunction in Liver Disease

Interactions between the heart and the liver have been described for many years with the understanding of 2 important entities.[16] Cardiac cirrhosis or congestive hepatopathy is liver dysfunction consequent to right-sided heart failure. In contrast, progression of chronic liver diseases may impair cardiac function, something that has been termed latent cardiac dysfunction, or sometimes cirrhotic cardiomyopathy. Despite the similar-sounding terminology, it is important to distinguish the two.

Cardiac Cirrhosis

The recognition and diagnosis of congestive hepatopathy caused by heart failure is important, because recovery of liver function relies predominantly on optimizing cardiac performance. The key mechanism underlying cardiac cirrhosis is passive congestion secondary to increased right ventricular filling pressures.[16]

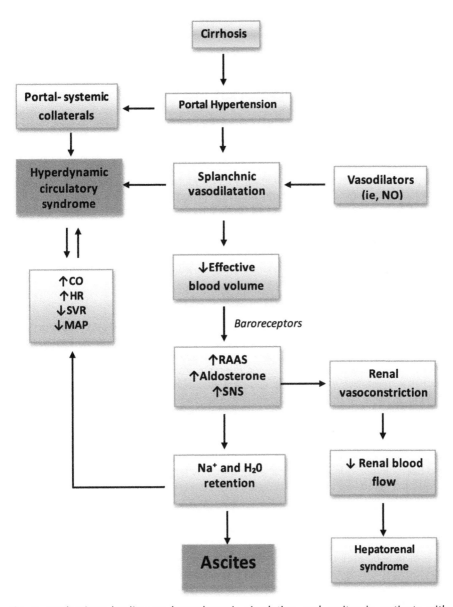

Fig. 1. Mechanisms leading to hyperdynamic circulation and ascites in patients with cirrhosis. In cirrhosis, portal hypertension leads to formation of portosystemic collaterals and splanchnic arterial vasodilatation. Increased circulating vasodilators such as NO are in part responsible for the arterial vasodilatation that occurs in both systemic and splanchnic circulations, leading to a hyperdynamic circulatory syndrome; increased CO and heart rate (HR); and decreased SVR, and mean arterial pressure (MAP). Abnormally distributed blood volume leads to increased baroreceptor-mediated activation of neurohormonal pathways such as the RAAS and SNS. As a result, increased sodium and water retention contributes to ascites and exacerbates the hyperdynamic circulatory state. Increased activation of RAAS and SNS also decreases renal blood flow and can lead to the development of hepatorenal syndrome. cAMP, cyclic AMP; TNF, tumor necrosis factor.

Right heart failure leading to congestive hepatopathy is characterized by edema, ascites, and hepatomegaly. Laboratory values generally reveal cholestasis with increased alkaline phosphatase and bilirubin levels, whereas transaminase levels may only be mildly increased. The severity of right heart failure can be assessed with echocardiography by evaluating the size and function of the right heart chambers. Pulmonary artery systolic pressure can also be calculated by using the tricuspid regurgitation jet velocity (V) to measure the right ventricle/right atrium systolic pressure gradient [$\Delta P = 4(V)^2$] and adding estimated right atrial pressure.[17]

Latent Cardiac Dysfunction

Cardiovascular dysfunction in patients with liver disease has been described for several decades, but for many years it was attributed to alcoholic cardiomyopathy. Because of the high CO in patients with cirrhosis, many clinicians assumed cardiac function to be normal. Over the last 20 years, it has been shown that cardiac dysfunction exists in nonalcoholic cirrhotic patients without known cardiac disease and may even precede complications such as hepatorenal syndrome.[18] Despite hyperdynamic circulation at rest, studies have shown a blunted cardiac response to stress or exercise that suggest unmasking of latent cardiac dysfunction.[19] This syndrome, termed cirrhotic cardiomyopathy, is summarized in **Box 2**.

Systolic Dysfunction

Hyperdynamic circulation in cirrhosis could lead to the assumption that cardiac function is normal in cirrhotic patients.[20] Left ventricular systolic function, as assessed by left ventricular ejection fraction (LVEF), has been shown to be normal (LVEF $\geq$ 55%) in most cirrhotic patients at rest. However, during exercise or stress, when left ventricular function is normally hyperdynamic, an attenuated increase in LVEF has been observed in patients with cirrhosis compared with matched controls.[21,22] The decrease in cardiac contractility is a result of reduced myocardial reserve, which is a measure of the difference between resting and maximum CO. Thus, if cardiac function is increased at baseline and the maximum response remains the same, then by definition the cardiac reserve will be decreased. A blunted heart rate response to exercise has also been observed in cirrhotic patients, and may further contribute to a reduction in cardiac performance, because CO is the product of heart rate and stroke volume.[21,22]

Left Ventricular Hypertrophy

Despite a decrease in cardiac afterload, left ventricular hypertrophy occurs in up to 30% of patients with advanced liver disease.[23] This hypertrophic response in cirrhotic patients may be attributable to hemodynamic overload (mechanical stress) or activation of neurohormonal pathways leading to cardiac remodeling and fibrosis.[24] Note that rapid regression of left ventricular hypertrophy occurs following liver transplant.[25]

Box 2
Characteristics of cirrhotic cardiomyopathy

- Impaired left ventricular systolic function with stress
- Absence of other known cardiac disease before diagnosis of liver failure
- Left ventricular hypertrophy
- Left ventricular diastolic dysfunction
- Electrophysiologic abnormalities

This regression of cardiomyocyte hypertrophy may be caused by alleviation of mechanical stress or reduced activation of RAAS and SNS.

Diastolic Dysfunction

In cirrhosis, myocardial hypertrophy and stiffening decreases left ventricular diastolic compliance. Therefore, small increases in intravascular volume can translate into significantly increased diastolic pressures. This effect was shown in one study in which left ventricular diastolic dysfunction, as assessed by the E wave/A wave ratio, was markedly worsened in the presence of tense ascites and improved following rapid, large-volume paracentesis.[26] Left ventricular diastolic dysfunction seems to be the earliest manifestation of cardiac disease in patients with cirrhotic cardiomyopathy, and has been found in up to 56% of patients using tissue Doppler echocardiography.[16,27] Diastolic dysfunction may also relate to a worse prognosis; the severity of diastolic dysfunction had a positive correlation with the degree of liver failure at 2-year follow-up.[26,28]

Electrophysiologic Abnormalities

Prolongation of the QT interval on the electrocardiogram is well documented in patients with cirrhosis, and may be caused by changes in plasma membrane fluidity and impairment of potassium ion channels.[21,29] QT prolongation potentially leads to ventricular arrhythmias and sudden cardiac death.[30] Moreover, QT prolongation is related to the severity of liver failure and seems to normalize with improvement in liver function following liver transplant.[31–33]

Abnormal chronotropic responses to physiologic and pharmacologic stimuli have also been observed in cirrhotic patients. Although many patients with cirrhosis are tachycardic, a failure to increase the heart rate further under certain physiologic states (ie, sepsis) may impair the ability of the heart to maintain an appropriate CO for the systemic demands.[34]

Pathophysiology of Cirrhotic Cardiomyopathy

The pathogenesis of cardiac dysfunction in liver disease is multifactorial. Several mechanisms have been proposed, many studied in cirrhotic rat models. These mechanisms include β-adrenergic receptor dysfunction, decreased fluidity of cardiomyocyte plasma membrane, and ion channel defects. Many of these defects in the cardiomyocyte result from increased activity of cardiodepressant substances such as cytokines, endogenous cannabinoids, and NO. See **Fig. 2** for a summary of the proposed cellular abnormalities in cirrhotic cardiomyopathy.

Clinical Impacts of Cardiac Dysfunction in Liver Disease

Despite a hyperdynamic circulatory state, many patients with cirrhosis decompensate under conditions that challenge the cardiovascular system; conditions that may be partly caused or worsened by cirrhotic cardiomyopathy. As liver function declines, cirrhotic patients often develop refractory ascites, infection, or variceal bleeding and may require interventions such as placement of a transjugular intrahepatic portosystemic shunt (TIPS) or, if a candidate, liver transplant. Patients with cirrhotic cardiomyopathy may respond poorly to these procedures and other forms of stress, such as infection caused by abrupt alterations in cardiac hemodynamics. In particular, liver transplant is associated with a high incidence of postoperative cardiovascular complications, including heart failure, arrhythmias, or myocardial infarction. Once the new liver is implanted, a reduction in the abnormal levels of circulating vasoactive substances occurs, decreasing the vasodilatory state that engenders hyperdynamic

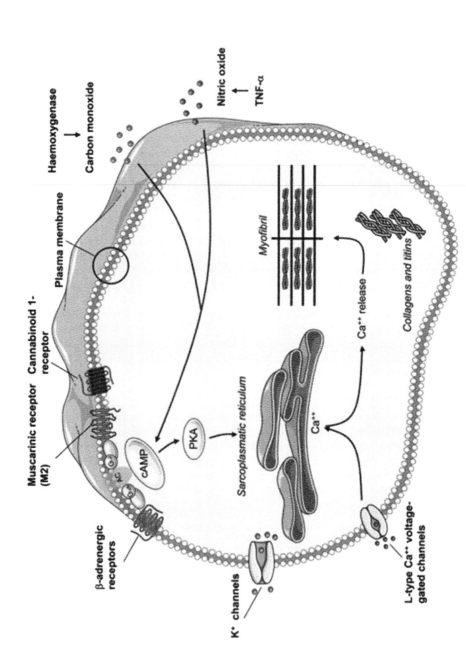

circulation.[16,35] However, the resulting increase in SVR and cardiac afterload, along with excessive fluid administration during surgery, may cause pulmonary edema or overt heart failure in the immediate postoperative period. Note that from 6 to 12 months after transplant, the hyperdynamic state resolves, diastolic function improves, and the systolic response to exercise and physical stress returns to normal, suggesting that cirrhotic cardiomyopathy is completely reversible with liver transplant.[19,25] QT interval prolongation in cirrhosis reverses following liver transplant as well.[32,33]

Unlike liver transplant, which reduces the high-output state, insertion of a TIPS has been shown to exacerbate the hyperdynamic circulatory state of cirrhotic patients because of a sudden increase in preload caused by the increased volume load shunted to the heart.[22,36,37] The onset of overt heart failure following placement of TIPS has been described, and is likely affected by the diastolic response to increased preload.[38] In one study, diastolic dysfunction was predictive of slow ascites clearance and increased mortality after TIPS placement.[22,39]

Hemodynamic Monitoring of Patients with Liver Disease in the Intensive Care Unit

More than 25,000 patients with cirrhosis require admission to the ICU each year in the United States, mostly because of infection (particularly spontaneous bacterial peritonitis), drug or alcoholic hepatitis, and gastrointestinal bleeding.[40] Intravascular volume assessments can be challenging in these patients, especially if latent cardiac dysfunction is present. For example, administration of intravenous fluid boluses to improve hypotension may abruptly increase preload in an already noncompliant ventricle that is unable to increase CO during stress, potentially worsening heart failure and hypotension. Measurement of central venous pressure (CVP) alone should not be used to make clinical decisions regarding fluid management, because left ventricular output is determined by left ventricular end-diastolic pressure and not right atrial pressure.[41] Moreover, patients with tense ascites or right-sided heart failure may have an increased CVP in the presence of volume depletion caused by increased intra-abdominal pressure or increased right heart pressures. In these situations, insertion of a pulmonary artery catheter may allow continuous hemodynamic monitoring of CO and pulmonary capillary wedge pressure to help guide titration of volume expanders, inotropes, or vasopressors.

When congestive heart failure predominates, treatment options are similar to those with noncirrhotic cardiac dysfunction with 1 important exception. Most patients with cirrhosis have low arterial blood pressures as a result of peripheral vasodilatation and therefore may not tolerate drugs that reduce preload or afterload.[20] Inotropic drugs such as dobutamine and milrinone may induce a precipitous decrease in blood

---

Fig. 2. A cardiomyocyte, showing the proposed abnormalities that are involved in the pathogenesis of cirrhotic cardiomyopathy. (1) Altered Ca^+ influx through L-type voltage-gated Ca^+ channels. (2) Reduced density of K^+ channels. (3) Decreased β-adrenergic receptor density or function may contribute to impaired inotropic and chronotropic response to stress. (4) Defective signal transduction of M2 muscarinic receptors to cAMP. (5) Upregulation of cannabinoid-1–receptor stimulation may induce arterial splanchnic vasodilatation and produce negative inotropic effects. (6) Altered plasma membrane cholesterol/phospholipid ratio may decrease plasma membrane fluidity, resulting in decreased cAMP production. (7) Upregulation of heme oxygenase in cirrhotic rats increases production of carbon monoxide, which may decrease ventricular contractility. (8) Increased levels of TNF-alpha stimulates NO production. (9) Altered ratio and function of collagens and titins. AC, adenylcyclase; G, G-protein; PKA, protein kinase A. (*Reproduced from* Møller S, Bernardi M. Interactions of the heart and the liver. Eur Heart J 2013;34:2807; with permission.)

pressure by causing further vasodilatation. The response to dobutamine may also be blunted in patients with cirrhosis. Thus norepinephrine, a potent vasoconstrictor with some inotropic effect, may be preferred when treating patients with cardiogenic shock and hypotension, especially in cirrhotic patients. Nonetheless, managing critically ill patients with cirrhosis and cardiac dysfunction may be challenging and often requires a multidisciplinary team approach.[40]

REFERENCES

1. Bolognesi M, Di Pascoli M, Verardo A, et al. Splanchnic vasodilation and hyperdynamic circulatory syndrome in cirrhosis. World J Gastroenterol 2014;20(10): 2555–63.
2. Feldman M, Friedman LS, Brandt LJ. Sleisenger and Fordtran's gastrointestinal and liver disease. 10th edition. Philadelphia: Saunders; 2016.
3. Licata A, Mazzola A, Ingrassia D. Clinical implications of the hyperdynamic syndrome in cirrhosis. Eur J Intern Med 2014;25(9):795–802.
4. Møller S, Bendtsen F, Henriksen JH. Effect of volume expansion on systemic hemodynamics and central and arterial blood volume in cirrhosis. Gastroenterology 1995;109(6):1917–25.
5. Iwakiri Y, Groszmann RJ. The hyperdynamic circulation of chronic liver diseases: from the patient to the molecule. Hepatology 2006;43:121–31.
6. Garcia-Tsao G, Bosch J. Management of varices and variceal hemorrhage in cirrhosis. N Engl J Med 2011;362(9):823–32.
7. Pârvu AE, Negrean V, Pleşca-Manea L, et al. Nitric oxide in patients with chronic liver diseases. Rom J Gastroenterol 2005;14(3):225–30.
8. El-Sherif M, Abou-Shady MA, Al-Bahrawy AM, et al. Nitric oxide levels in chronic liver disease patients with and without esophageal varices. Hepatol Int 2008;2: 341–5.
9. Fernandez M, Vizzutti F, Garcia-Pagan JC, et al. Anti-VEGF receptor-2 monoclonal antibody prevents portal-systemic collateral vessel formation in portal hypertensive mice. Gastroenterology 2004;126(3):886–94.
10. Kashani A, Landaverde C, Medici V, et al. Fluid retention in cirrhosis: pathophysiology and management. QJM 2008;101(2):71–85.
11. Planas R, Montoliu S, Ballesté B, et al. Natural history of patients hospitalized for management of cirrhotic ascites. Clin Gastroenterol Hepatol 2006;4(11):1385–94.
12. Moore KP, Wong F, Gines P, et al. The management of ascites in cirrhosis: report on the consensus conference of the International Ascites Club. Hepatology 2003; 38(1):258–66.
13. Reynolds TB. Ascites. Clin Liver Dis 2000;4(1):151–68.
14. Runyon BA, Montano AA, Akriviadis EA, et al. The serum-ascites albumin gradient is superior to the exudate-transudate concept in the differential diagnosis of ascites. Ann Intern Med 1992;117:215–20.
15. Hou W, Sanyal AJ. Ascites: diagnosis and management. Med Clin North Am 2009;93(4):801–17, vii.
16. Møller S, Bernardi M. Interactions of the heart and the liver. Eur Heart J 2013;34: 2804–11.
17. Otto CM, Schwaegler RG, Freeman RV. Echocardiography review guide. 2nd edition. Philadelphia: Elsevier; 2011.
18. Krag A, Bendtsen F, Burroughs AK, et al. The cardiorenal link in advanced cirrhosis. Med Hypotheses 2012;79(1):53–5.

19. Yang YY, Lin H-C. The heart: pathophysiology and clinical implications of cirrhotic cardiomyopathy. J Chin Med Assoc 2012;75:619–23.
20. Lee RF, Glenn TK, Lee SS. Cardiac dysfunction in cirrhosis. Best Pract Res Clin Gastroenterol 2007;21(1):125–40.
21. Møller S, Henriksen JH. Cirrhotic cardiomyopathy a pathophysiological review of circulatory dysfunction in liver disease. Heart 2002;87:9–15.
22. Fede G, Privitera G, Tomaselli T, et al. Cardiovascular dysfunction in patients with liver cirrhosis. Ann Gastroenterol 2015;28(1):31–40.
23. Batra S, Machicao VI, Bynon JS, et al, Pulmonary Vascular Complications of Liver Disease Group. The impact of left ventricular hypertrophy on survival in candidates for liver transplantation. Liver Transpl 2014;20(6):705–12.
24. De Marco M, Chinali M, Romano C, et al. Increased left ventricular mass in pre-liver transplantation cirrhotic patients. J Cardiovasc Med (Hagerstown) 2008;9(2):142–6.
25. Torregrosa M, Aguadé S, Dos L, et al. Cardiac alterations in cirrhosis: reversibility after liver transplantation. J Hepatol 2005;42(1):68–74.
26. Pozzi M, Carugo S, Boari G, et al. Evidence of functional and structural cardiac abnormalities in cirrhotic patients with and without ascites. Hepatology 1997; 26(5):1131–7.
27. Wong F, Villamil A, Merli M, et al. Prevalence of diastolic dysfunction in cirrhosis and its clinical significance. Hepatology 2011;54(Suppl 1):A475–6.
28. Karagiannakis DS, Vlachogiannakos J, Anastasiadis G, et al. Diastolic cardiac dysfunction is a predictor of dismal prognosis in patients with liver cirrhosis. Hepatol Int 2014;8:588–94.
29. Ward CA, Ma Z, Lee SS, et al. Potassium currents in atrial and ventricular myocytes from a rat model of cirrhosis. Am J Physiol Gastrointest Liver Physiol 1997;273(2):537–44.
30. Day CP, James OF, Butler TJ, et al. QT prolongation and sudden cardiac death in patients with alcoholic liver disease. Lancet 1993;341(8858):1423–8.
31. Bernardi M, Calandra S, Colantoni A, et al. Q-T interval prolongation in cirrhosis: prevalence, relationship with severity, and etiology of the disease and possible pathogenetic factors. Hepatology 1998;27(1):28–34.
32. Mohamed R, Forsey PR, Davies MK, et al. Effect of liver transplantation on QT interval prolongation and autonomic dysfunction in end-stage liver disease. Hepatology 1996;23(5):1128–34.
33. García González M, Hernandez-Madrid A, Lopez-Sanromán A, et al. Reversal of QT interval electrocardiographic alterations in cirrhotic patients undergoing liver transplantation. Transplant Proc 1999;31(6):2366–77.
34. Zambruni A, Trevisani F, Caraceni P, et al. Cardiac electrophysiological abnormalities in patients with cirrhosis. J Hepatol 2006;44(5):994–1002.
35. Therapondos G, Flapan AD, Plevris JN, et al. Cardiac morbidity and mortality related to orthotopic liver transplantation. Liver Transpl 2004;10:1441–53.
36. Azoulay D, Castaing D, Dennison A, et al. Transjugular intrahepatic portosystemic shunt worsens the hyperdynamic circulatory state of the cirrhotic patient: preliminary report of a prospective study. Hepatology 1994;19(1):129–32.
37. Merli M, Valeriano V, Funaro S, et al. Modifications of cardiac function in cirrhotic patients treated with transjugular intrahepatic portosystemic shunt (TIPS). Am J Gastroenterol 2002;97(1):142–8.
38. Braverman AC, Steiner MA, Picus D, et al. High-output congestive heart failure following transjugular intrahepatic portal-systemic shunting. Chest 1995;107: 1467–9.

39. Rabie RN, Cazzaniga M, Salerno F, et al. The use of E/A ratio as a predictor of outcome in cirrhotic patients treated with transjugular intrahepatic portosystemic shunt. Am J Gastroenterol 2009;104:2458–66.
40. Olson JC, Wendon JA, Kramer DJ, et al. Intensive care of the patient with cirrhosis. Hepatology 2011;54(5):1864–72.
41. Marik PE, Baram M, Vahid B. Does central venous pressure predict fluid responsiveness? A systematic review of the literature and the tale of seven mares. Chest 2008;134(1):172–8.

Kidney Injury in Liver Disease

Kevin R. Regner, MD, MS[a], Kai Singbartl, MD, MPH[b],*

KEYWORDS

- Acute kidney injury • Cirrhosis • Liver transplant • Hepatorenal syndrome

KEY POINTS

- Acute kidney injury (AKI) occurs frequently in patients with liver disease and increases morbidity and mortality.
- Hepatorenal syndrome (HRS) is a common cause of AKI in patients with decompensated cirrhosis and is due to alterations in systemic and renal hemodynamics.
- Serum creatinine based estimation of kidney function is a key component of the Model for End-stage Liver Disease score in liver transplant candidates.
- Continuous renal replacement therapy is used in critically ill patients with liver failure and AKI.
- Simultaneous liver–kidney transplantation (SLK) may be required in patients with liver failure and prolonged AKI. Identification of appropriate candidates for SLK remains controversial.

DEFINITION OF ACUTE KIDNEY INJURY

Acute kidney injury (AKI) describes the abrupt decrease in renal function. AKI represents a broad clinical syndrome that entails numerous etiologies, which are classified by their location into prerenal, intrarenal, and postrenal. Hypovolemia, acute tubular necrosis, acute interstitial nephritis, acute glomerular diseases, and acute obstructive nephropathies represent the most common underlying causes. Established consensus criteria rely on only 2 easily obtainable clinical variables to diagnose and stage AKI, namely, (changes in) serum creatinine and urine output (**Fig. 1**).[1–3]

AKI continues to be a serious clinical challenge that carries high morbidity and mortality rates. Depending on its severity, AKI is associated with a 2- to 6-fold increase in

Disclosure: The authors have no commercial or financial conflicts to disclose. K.R. Regner is supported by grants DK90123 and DK098104 from the NIH and 5520353 from Advancing a Healthier Wisconsin.
[a] Division of Nephrology, Medical College of Wisconsin, 9200 West Wisconsin Avenue, Milwaukee, WI 53226, USA; [b] Department of Anesthesiology, Milton S. Hershey Medical Center, Penn State College of Medicine, PO Box 850, H187, Hershey, PA 17033, USA
* Corresponding author.
E-mail address: ksingbartl@hmc.psu.edu

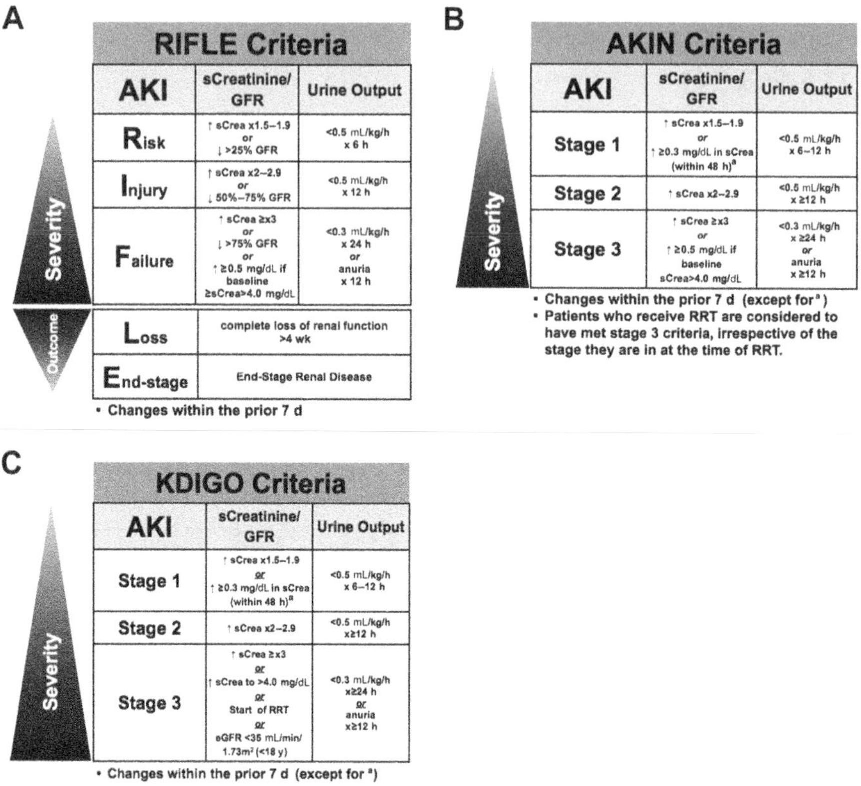

A

B

C

Fig. 1. Direct comparison of (A) risk of renal dysfunction, injury to the kidney, failure or loss of kidney function, and end-stage kidney disease (RIFLE),[1] (B) ACUTE KIDNEY INJURY NETWORK (AKIN)[2] and (C) kidney disease: improving global outcomes (KDIGO) foundation criteria[3] to classify AKI. GFR, glomerular filtration rate; RRT, renal replacement therapy; sCREA, serum creatinine. (Data from Refs.[1–3])

risk of death.[4] AKI at all stages also negatively affects duration of hospital stay, readmission rates, and development of chronic kidney disease. The clinical presentation of AKI is the same regardless of the underlying etiology.

EPIDEMIOLOGY AND ETIOLOGY OF ACUTE KIDNEY INJURY IN LIVER DISEASE
Acute Kidney Injury and Acute Liver Failure

AKI develops in up to 80% of patients with acute liver failure (ALF).[5,6] Approximately 30% to 50% of these patients will require renal replacement therapy (RRT). The majority of AKI cases occur in patients with ALF owing to ischemic hepatitis or acetaminophen intoxication. These patients also require RRT more often than patients with other etiologies of ALF. Irrespective of the underlying etiology, AKI represents a crucial risk factor that significantly lowers the rate of spontaneous survival. The need for RRT further decreases transplant-free survival rates in patients with ALF. However, fewer than 5% of the survivors develop end-stage renal disease and require long-term dialysis.

The etiology of underlying AKI in patients with ALF is often multifactorial and encompasses insults also seen in the general AKI population, for example, sepsis, nephrotoxins, ischemia/hypoperfusion, and hypovolemia.[4]

Because acetaminophen also exerts direct nephrotoxic effects and remains the number one cause for ALF in the United States, it is not surprising that it is also the most frequent cause for AKI in patients with ALF. Although strong clinical data are missing, available small case series and animal data suggest that the features of acetaminophen-induced kidney injury resemble those seen in acute tubular necrosis.[7–9] Here, characteristic urine sediment and elevated urine sodium levels are hallmarks of acetaminophen-induced AKI. These findings allow one to distinguish acetaminophen-induced AKI from the hepatorenal syndrome (HRS), a prerenal form of AKI in patients with chronic liver disease.

Because of its similarity with AKI in the general population, management and treatment options for AKI in patients with ALF are also identical to those in the general population.[4] Options for RRT in these patients will be discussed further elsewhere in this article.

Acute Kidney Injury and Chronic Liver Disease

In patients with CLD, such as cirrhosis, AKI occurs frequently and remains a major clinical problem with devastating complications. Nearly 20% of patients hospitalized with cirrhosis develop AKI and mortality rates as high as 50% to 90% have been reported.[10–14]

More than 60% of all AKI cases in patients with cirrhosis are attributable to prerenal factors, for example, hypovolemia, hypoperfusion. Intrarenal causes, for example, acute tubular necrosis and acute glomerular pathologies, account for at least 30% of all AKI cases in patients with cirrhosis. Fewer than 1% of all AKI cases in patients with cirrhosis have been found to be owing to acute obstructive nephropathies.[15]

HRS is a very distinct form of AKI in patients with CLD. HRS is the consequence of massive renal vasoconstriction in the setting of systemic and splanchnic arterial vasodilation. HRS is considered a prerenal kidney insult and occurs in approximately 20% of all AKI cases in patients hospitalized with cirrhosis. Because of its unique features with respect to diagnosis, management and prognosis, HRS will be discussed more extensively elsewhere in this paper.

Non-HRS cases of AKI in patients with CLD follow a similar approach for diagnosis and management as AKI in the general patient population.

ASSESSING KIDNEY FUNCTION IN LIVER DISEASE

Accurate assessments of renal function continue to be difficult in critically ill patients, especially in those with underlying liver disease. Serum creatinine measurements have been the gold standard for assessment of renal function for decades. Moreover, serum creatinine is also an important prognostic marker in patients with end-stage liver disease. Serum creatinine is 1 of 4 variables that serve to calculate the Model for End-stage Liver Disease score, which in turn plays a crucial role in prioritizing patients for liver transplantation (LT). Despite its widespread use, serum creatinine as a biomarker of kidney function has several limitations.

Serum creatinine greatly depends on body weight, race, age and gender. CLD further hinders accurate assessment of renal function in these patients because of the following disease-specific factors: (A) malnutrition, muscle wasting and impaired liver function all lead to a decreased creatinine production, (B) some laboratory assays (Jaffé reaction-based) will give falsely low serum creatinine concentrations in the setting of high bilirubin levels, (C) increased secretion of creatinine by renal tubular cells, and (D) dilution of serum creatinine owing to an expanded volume of distribution.[16]

Use of serum creatinine in patients with CLD consequently carries the risk of overestimating renal function (glomerular filtration rate [GFR]). For example, a "normal" serum creatinine (<1.0 mg/dL) has been associated with a wide range of measured GFR (34–163 mL/min/1.73 m²) in patients with cirrhosis. Overestimation of renal function can result in a lower priority for LT in patients with a truly low GFR but still "normal" serum creatinine.[17]

The limitations of serum creatinine as a marker of renal function, not only in patients with CLD, have stimulated intense research efforts to find better alternatives. Serum cystatin C has emerged as a promising alternative among the various biomarkers studied in patients with CLD.[18,19] However, cystatin C is also affected by age, gender, muscle mass, and liver function. It likewise tends to overestimate GFR. Measurements of serum cystatin C overall do not seem to be superior clinically to measurements of serum creatinine. However, GFR formulas based on serum cystatin C seem to be more accurate than traditional formulas (eg, Modification of Diet in Renal Disease [MDRD] equation) that are based on serum creatinine.

To this end, serum creatinine remains the only established marker of renal function in patients with CLD. The use of serum creatinine to assess renal function in patients with CLD, however, requires a careful approach and consideration of the following caveats:

- Serum creatinine is a poor reflection of an individual patient's true renal function.
- Serum creatinine tends to overestimate the true renal function.
- The use of only 1 measurement (static threshold) to assess the patient's status and prognosis does not consider the dynamic and complex nature of renal function in patients with CLD.

DIAGNOSING AND STAGING ACUTE RENAL (DYS-) FUNCTION AND INJURY IN LIVER DISEASE

The difficulty in diagnosing and staging renal dysfunction and injury is not unique to patients with CLD and has been a longstanding challenge in a variety of clinical situations. Presumably, the most critical obstacle to improve the care of patients with renal injury was the lack of well-accepted and validated consensus definitions to diagnose and stage AKI.[4]

The Acute Dialysis Quality Initiative made the first attempt to overcome this problem (see **Fig. 1**A).[1] The group developed the Risk, Injury, Failure; Loss and End-stage kidney disease (RIFLE system) to diagnose and stage acute impairment of renal function through broad consensus among several international experts. The RIFLE classification is based on 2 common and easily obtainable clinical variables: changes in serum creatinine and urine output. The RIFLE criteria have been evaluated in more than 1 million patients as of to date and have been proven to be an excellent predictor of outcome. In patients developing AKI, the risk of death increases with the severity of renal injury, from 2.4-fold for RIFLE-R to more than 6-fold for RIFLE-F.[4]

The Acute Kidney Injury Network proposed a modification to the RIFLE criteria to include small changes in serum creatinine occurring within a 48-hour period (see **Fig. 1**B).[2] Analyses of 2 large databases in both Europe and the United States have found these modifications to be valid.[3]

Despite great efforts, inconsistent application of criteria and determination of baseline serum creatinine values have continued to be problematic and subsequently prompted the formulation of unified and more precise criteria to diagnose and stage AKI. The Kidney Disease: Improving Global Outcomes foundation has developed and published the first international, interdisciplinary clinical guideline on AKI to be used for clinical practice, research and public health efforts (see **Fig. 1C**).[3]

Several studies have validated RIFLE or Acute Kidney Injury Network criteria in patients with CLD.[10,12,20–22] All studies found that the development of AKI as diagnosed by either set of criteria was independently associated with an increase in mortality, often in a stage-dependent manner. Moreover, AKI severity frequently progresses in cirrhotic patients after admission to the intensive care unit (ICU).

Several features unique to patients with CLD/cirrhosis have raised concerns regarding the application of any general AKI classification scheme of modifications.[23] In particular, the use of urine output as a criterion has been deemed inappropriate. Many CLD patients have preserved GFR despite ongoing oliguria. Consideration of these concerns has led the International Club of Ascites to develop new guidelines for diagnosing, staging, and managing AKI in patients with cirrhosis (**Fig. 2**).[23]

In addition to a standardized approach to staging and diagnosing AKI, all classification schemes also offer the potential to diagnose AKI earlier (in patients with CLD), expanding the time window for preventive and/or therapeutic interventions.

HEPATORENAL SYNDROME
Epidemiology and Etiology

HRS occurs in approximately 20% of patients with advanced cirrhosis during the first year after diagnosis, and in up to 40% during the first 5 years after diagnosis. Alterations in systemic and renal hemodynamics play key roles in the pathophysiology of HRS. Patients with liver cirrhosis develop severe splanchnic arterial vasodilation. In compensated liver cirrhosis, this is accompanied by an increase in cardiac output and plasma volume, preserving the effective arterial blood volume.[24,25] In decompensated liver cirrhosis, however, simultaneously developing cirrhotic cardiomyopathy impairs the compensatory increase in cardiac output. Consequently, the effective arterial blood volume decreases, causing activation of Na^+-retaining and vasoconstrictor systems. Subsequent Na^+ and water retention lead to ascites formation.

ICA-AKI Criteria

AKI	sCreatinine/ GFR	Urine Output
Stage 1	↑ sCrea x1.5–2.0 *or* ↑ ≥0.3 mg/dL in sCrea (within 48 h)[a]	N/A
Stage 2	↑ sCrea >x2 to x3	N/A
Stage 3	↑ sCrea >x3 *or* ↑ sCrea to >4.0 mg/dL *or* Start of RRT	N/A

Severity

- Changes within the prior 7 d (except for [a])
- Response to treatment:
  · No response - No regression of AKI
  · Partial response - Regression of AKI stage (sCr remains ↑ ≥0.3 mg/dL from baseline)
  · Full response - sCr ↑ <0.3 mg/dL from baseline

Fig. 2. International Club of Ascites Acute Kidney Injury (ICA-AKI) new definitions for the diagnosis of AKI in patients with cirrhosis.[23] Contrary to other classifications, urine output has been deemed an unreliable and even misleading criterion to diagnose AKI in patients with cirrhosis. ICA-AKI criteria therefore solely rely on changes in serum creatinine for staging and diagnosing. RRT, renal replacement therapy; sCREA, serum creatinine.

Ascites formation triggers further activation of vasoconstrictor systems. Any additional insult in this situation, for example, infection, will precipitate a further decrease in cardiac output, leading to overwhelming intrarenal vasoconstriction and ultimately decreased GFR. Decreasing GFR will manifest itself eventually by a (delayed) increase in serum creatinine, originally termed HRS.[24,25]

Definition and Diagnosis

Besides a serum creatinine greater than 1.5 mg/dL or 24-hour creatinine clearance of less than 40 mL/min, HRS is largely a diagnosis by exclusion (**Box 1**).[26] It became apparent over time that the proposed criteria were too restrictive. For example, an ongoing bacterial infection was considered an exclusion criterion, although bacterial infections are frequently seen as a clinical trigger for HRS.[24,25] According to the original definition, cirrhotic patients with diabetic nephropathy also cannot develop HRS, because they have underlying parenchymal renal disease. The definition of HRS was revised approximately 10 years later. Some of the original exclusion criteria, for example, bacterial infection, were removed, but evidence of preexisting parenchymal kidney disease remained an exclusion criterion.[27] Both definitions also continue to rely on one single (static) serum creatinine value.

Traditionally, 2 forms of HRS have been described, based on presentation and severity.[23,26,27]

- *Type I HRS*: an abrupt, rapid increase in serum creatinine (<2 weeks, >100% of baseline, >2.5 mg/dL); untreated median survival is less than 2 weeks.
- *Type II HRS:* slower, less severe increase in serum creatinine (>2 weeks, 1.5 mg/dL > serum creatinine <2.5 mg/dL); untreated median survival is 4 to 6 months.

Box 1
International Ascites Club's diagnostic criteria of hepatorenal syndrome

Major Criteria

- Chronic or acute liver disease with advanced hepatic failure and portal hypertension.
- Low glomerular filtration rate, as indicated by serum creatinine of greater than 1.5 mg/dL or 24-h creatinine clearance of less than 40 mL/min.
- Absence of shock, ongoing bacterial infection, and current or recent treatment with nephrotoxic drugs. Absence of gastrointestinal fluid losses (repeated vomiting or intense diarrhea) or renal fluid losses (weight loss >500 g/d for several days in patients with ascites without peripheral edema or 1000 g/d in patients with peripheral edema).
- No sustained improvement in renal function (decrease in serum creatinine to 1.5 mg/dL or less or increase in creatinine clearance to 40 mL/min or more) after diuretic withdrawal and expansion of plasma volume with 1.5 L of isotonic saline.
- Proteinuria less than 500 mg/dL and no ultrasonographic evidence of obstructive uropathy or parenchymal renal disease.

Additional criteria

- Urine volume less than 500 mL/d.
- Urine Na^+ of less than 10 mmol/L. Urine osmolality greater than plasma osmolality.
- Urine red blood cells less than 50 per high-power field.
- Serum Na^+ concentration of less than 130 mmol/L.

Adapted from Arroyo V, Gines P, Gerbes A, et al. Definition and diagnostic criteria of refractory ascites and hepatorenal syndrome in cirrhosis. Hepatology 1996;23:165.

Patients with type I HRS will also meet criteria for stage 2 AKI. Here, the introduction and acceptance of easily applicable criteria to diagnose and stage AKI hold great promise for earlier detection of evolving HRS type I in the future. HRS type I should be included in the differential diagnoses in any patient with CLD presenting with AKI.

Management of Patients with the Hepatorenal Syndrome

Compared with many other forms of AKI, reversal of type I HRS is possible and can improve short-term mortality.[28–33] In ICU patients, the mainstays for type I HRS treatment are the appropriate use of colloids and vasopressors to restore effective blood volume and maintain sufficient perfusion pressure.[28–33]

There is no clinical evidence supporting the preference for one vasopressor over another. All currently available vasopressors, that is, vasopressin, norepinephrine, or terlipressin, are effective in raising blood pressure. The goal is to raise the mean arterial blood pressure by at least 10 mm Hg from baseline or to an absolute value of greater than 70 mm Hg. Volume expansion with a hyperoncotic colloid, for example, albumin 20%, should occur simultaneously. Albumin 20% is initially administered at 1 g/kg per day for 2 days, with a maximum of 100 g/d, and then followed by 20 to 40 g/d.

Neither treatment with vasopressors nor treatment with colloids alone is effective in reversing HRS type I. There is some clinical evidence supporting the use of albumin and vasopressors to also reverse type II HRS. The limited number of patients studied, however, precludes the formulation of general treatment recommendations.

METABOLIC ACIDOSIS IN LIVER DISEASE
Etiology

Metabolic acidosis (MA) frequently complicates AKI in patients with liver disease and may also occur in the setting of preserved renal function. The major causes of MA in critically ill patients with liver disease include anion gap MA (lactic acidosis, ketoacidosis) and non–anion gap metabolic acidosis (diarrhea, renal tubular acidosis).

Anion gap metabolic acidosis
Lactic acidosis Type A lactic acidosis (LA) occurs in response to tissue hypoperfusion, leading to an increase in anaerobic glycolysis and frequently occurs in patients with decompensated liver disease, especially in the setting of sepsis or hemorrhage.[34,35] Type B LA may occur in the absence of tissue hypoperfusion. In this setting, lactate production is normal, but lactate use is decreased owing to liver dysfunction.[34,35]

Ketoacidosis Alcoholic ketoacidosis (KA) may present in patients with CLD in response to reduced caloric intake and/or volume depletion owing to vomiting after an episode of binge drinking. Hepatic oxidation of ethanol yields acetaldehyde, which is ultimately converted into the ketone bodies acetoacetic acid and β-hydroxybutyrate leading to anion gap MA.[36]

Non–anion gap metabolic acidosis
Diarrhea In patients with liver disease, lactulose therapy for hepatic encephalopathy can produce diarrhea and stool bicarbonate loss leading to MA.[34]

Renal tubular acidosis Renal tubular acidosis (RTA) occurs owing to the failure of the kidneys to excrete the daily acid load. In patients with CLD, distal RTA can result from an intrinsic distal tubular acidification defect associated with autoimmune disease (eg, primary biliary cirrhosis).[34,37] Alternatively, decreased effective circulating volume owing to liver failure leads to impaired distal tubule sodium delivery and an impairment of distal tubular acidification. In this setting, the distal tubular acidification defect resolves when distal sodium delivery increases.[34]

Diagnosis

The evaluation of MA in patients with liver disease is similar to that of other critically ill patients. The presence of an anion gap MA should prompt investigation for LA, KA, methanol or ethylene glycol ingestion, or salicylate ingestion. In patients with acetaminophen toxicity, MA owing to 5-oxoproline (or pyroglutamic acid) should be considered.[34,35,38] Sources of bicarbonate loss (eg, diarrhea) should be identified in cases of non–anion gap MA. In the absence of stool losses, distal RTA should be considered in patients with otherwise unexplained hyperchloremic MA. The urine anion gap will be positive in distal RTA, whereas diarrhea will be associated with a negative urine anion gap. However, the urine pH and urine anion gap should be interpreted with caution in the setting of urine sodium less than 25 mEq/L owing to the impact of distal sodium delivery on the capacity for urine acidification.[34]

Management

Treatment of MA is directed at the underlying cause. Optimization of systemic hemodynamics is the mainstay of treatment of type A LA. Discontinuation of offending medications (eg, metformin, nucleoside reverse-transcriptase inhibitors) may be necessary in cases of LA.[38] KA can be corrected by administration of dextrose- and saline-containing intravenous fluids. In alcoholic patients, thiamine administration may be necessary for treatment of LA owing to thiamine deficiency and/or for prevention of Wernicke–Korsakoff syndrome after treatment for KA.[36,38] In CLD patients with non–anion gap MA owing to diarrhea, lactulose therapy should be modified to decrease the frequency of loose stools. Alkali therapy with sodium bicarbonate may be necessary in cases of distal RTA or in severe, refractory LA but may be complicated by intracellular acidosis and/or worsening ascites and edema. In patients with concomitant AKI, refractory MA is an indication for the initiation of dialysis.[35,38]

RENAL REPLACEMENT THERAPY IN LIVER DISEASE
Indications for Renal Replacement Therapy and Patient Selection

In patients with liver failure and AKI, the indications for dialysis initiation are similar to those in other critically ill patients and include uremic signs and symptoms, hyperkalemia, volume overload, or refractory MA. Additional indications unique to this patient population include severe hyponatremia or volume overload leading to increased intracranial pressure and risk of brainstem herniation.[39,40]

In the setting of multiorgan failure, the decision to initiate RRT for AKI in patients with liver failure should be informed by the underlying cause of AKI and nonrenal prognostic factors.[39] In general, initiation of RRT for AKI is appropriate as a bridge to transplantation in patients who are liver transplant candidates. In patients who are not transplant candidates, frank discussions should be performed with all stakeholders, including the patient and family, before initiation of RRT. Because the underlying etiology of renal dysfunction in patients with liver failure is often unclear, a time limited trial of RRT can be performed to allow time for assessment of transplant candidacy and to assess for signs of renal recovery. Prolonged dialysis is not indicated in nontransplant candidates without evidence of renal recovery after this trial of supportive care and RRT.[39]

Renal Replacement Therapy Modalities

The primary RRT modalities for treatment of AKI in critically ill patients include intermittent hemodialysis or continuous RRT (CRRT).[40] CRRT is frequently the modality of choice in hemodynamically unstable patients in the ICU and offers several additional advantages in patients with liver failure. CRRT allows for the gradual correction of tonicity in patients with severe hyponatremia.[39,40] In contrast with intermittent hemodialysis, CRRT does not increase intracranial pressure and is therefore the treatment of choice in fulminant hepatic failure or during LT, settings where intracranial pressure is known to increase.[39]

An additional advantage of CRRT is the feasibility of providing RRT intraoperatively during LT.[41–43] Intraoperative CRRT can be performed as a continuation of pretransplant RRT or initiated at the time of LT. In either case, indications for intraoperative CRRT include control of preexisting volume overload or acid–base and electrolyte abnormalities or anticipation of large volume transfusions or life-threatening hyperkalemia upon liver allograft reperfusion.[40–43]

Complications of Renal Replacement Therapy

Patients with liver failure are at increased risk for several known complications of RRT. Bleeding owing to coagulopathy and thrombocytopenia can complicate venous access placement for RRT. Hemodynamic instability owing to ultrafiltration during RRT may be more profound in liver failure patients with compromised systemic hemodynamics owing to third spacing or hemorrhage. Anticoagulation of CRRT circuits is challenging in patients with liver failure. The risk of filter clotting and subsequent blood loss seems to be greater in these patients.[40] However, administration of systemic anticoagulants can exacerbate gastrointestinal bleeding and regional citrate anticoagulation can lead to ionized hypocalcemia and anion gap MA owing to impaired hepatic metabolism of citrate to bicarbonate.[40] Therefore, decisions regarding the use and method of anticoagulation should weigh the benefits of anticoagulation against these potential risks in a patient-specific manner.[42]

SIMULTANEOUS LIVER–KIDNEY TRANSPLANTATION
Outcomes

LT is the definitive treatment for liver failure and associated HRS. In patients with renal failure owing to HRS, renal function often improves after LT allowing discontinuation of RRT. However, renal recovery is insufficient in some LT patients leading to inferior posttransplant outcomes.[44] Therefore, simultaneous liver–kidney transplantation (SLK) has been increasingly used in LT candidates with prolonged AKI or chronic kidney disease.[44,45] In comparison with LT alone, SLK has been associated with a lesser risk of both graft loss and mortality in patients with pretransplant renal failure.[46–48]

Predictors of Renal Recovery after Liver Transplantation

Functional recovery of native kidneys occurs in some patients after SLK despite pretransplant predictions of irreversible kidney failure.[49] Therefore, more accurate methods to predict the likelihood of renal recovery after LT are needed to avoid unnecessary kidney transplantation in LT candidates and to optimize the benefit of donor kidneys for patients with end-stage renal disease.

Recovery of renal function seems to be higher after LT in female recipients and recipients with lower body mass index whereas diabetes and/or pretransplant estimated GFR less than 30 mL/min/1.73 m^2 are associated with a higher risk of end-stage renal disease.[50–52] Percutaneous renal biopsy can be used to establish the underlying cause of renal failure and predict renal prognosis in LT candidates. Patients with significant renal interstitial fibrosis or glomerulosclerosis upon kidney biopsy should proceed to SLK. Although biopsy findings can assist in patient selection for SLK, the

---

Box 2
Criteria for simultaneous liver–kidney transplantation

Candidates with persistent AKI for 4 weeks or more with 1 of the following:
- Increase in serum creatinine 3× baseline, serum creatinine 4.0 mg/dL or greater with an acute increase of 0.5 mg/dL or greater, or on RRT.
- eGFR of 35 mL/min or less (MDRD equation) or GFR of 25 mL/min or less (iothalamate clearance).

Candidates with CKD for 3 months with 1 of the following:
- eGFR of 40 mL/min of less (MDRD equation) or GFR of 30 mL/min or less (iothalamate clearance).
- Proteinuria 2 g/d or greater.
- Kidney biopsy with greater than 30% global glomerulosclerosis or greater than 30% interstitial fibrosis
- Metabolic disease (eg, diabetes)

Abbreviations: AKI, acute kidney injury; CKD, chronic kidney disease; eGFR, estimated glomerular filtration rate; GFR, glomerular filtration rate; MDRD, modification of diet in renal disease; RRT, renal replacement therapy.
Adapted from Nadim MK, Sung RS, Davis CL, et al. Simultaneous liver-kidney transplantation summit: current state and future directions. Am J Transplant 2012;12:2901–8.

---

benefit of Percutaneous renal biopsy should be weighed against the approximately 30% risk of complications (eg, retroperitoneal hematoma, gross hematuria), especially in patients with an International Normalized Ration of 1.5 or greater.[53] Radionuclide renal scans may provide a noninvasive method to assess native kidney function before transplant and could prove useful in predicting renal recovery after LT.[34]

Selection Criteria for Simultaneous Liver–Kidney Transplantation

The findings of a consensus summit on SLK were published in 2012 and include criteria for SLK in LT candidates with AKI and/or chronic kidney disease. These recommendations are summarized in **Box 2**.[44]

REFERENCES

1. Bellomo R, Ronco C, Kellum JA, et al. Acute renal failure - definition, outcome measures, animal models, fluid therapy and information technology needs: the Second International Consensus Conference of the Acute Dialysis Quality Initiative (ADQI) Group. Crit Care 2004;8:R204–12.

2. Ronco C, Levin A, Warnock DG, et al. Improving outcomes from acute kidney injury (AKI): report on an initiative. Int J Artif Organs 2007;30:373–6.

3. Kellum JA, Lameire N, KDIGO AKI Guideline Work Group. Diagnosis, evaluation, and management of acute kidney injury: a KDIGO summary (part 1). Crit Care 2013;17:204.

4. Singbartl K, Kellum JA. AKI in the ICU: definition, epidemiology, risk stratification, and outcomes. Kidney Int 2012;81:819–25.

5. Tujios SR, Hynan LS, Vazquez MA, et al. Risk factors and outcomes of acute kidney injury in patients with acute liver failure. Clin Gastroenterol Hepatol 2015;13: 352–9.

6. O'Riordan A, Brummell Z, Sizer E, et al. Acute kidney injury in patients admitted to a liver intensive therapy unit with paracetamol-induced hepatotoxicity. Nephrol Dial Transplant 2011;26:3501–8.

7. Blakely P, McDonald BR. Acute renal failure due to acetaminophen ingestion: a case report and review of the literature. J Am Soc Nephrol 1995;6:48–53.

8. Waring WS, Jamie H, Leggett GE. Delayed onset of acute renal failure after significant paracetamol overdose: a case series. Hum Exp Toxicol 2010;29:63–8.

9. Mazer M, Perrone J. Acetaminophen-induced nephrotoxicity: pathophysiology, clinical manifestations, and management. J Med Toxicol 2008;4:2–6.

10. Wong F, O'Leary JG, Reddy KR, et al. New consensus definition of acute kidney injury accurately predicts 30-day mortality in patients with cirrhosis and infection. Gastroenterology 2013;145:1280–8.e1.

11. de Carvalho JR, Villela-Nogueira CA, Luiz RR, et al. Acute Kidney Injury Network criteria as a predictor of hospital mortality in cirrhotic patients with ascites. J Clin Gastroenterol 2012;46:e21–6.

12. Fagundes C, Barreto R, Guevara M, et al. A modified acute kidney injury classification for diagnosis and risk stratification of impairment of kidney function in cirrhosis. J Hepatol 2013;59:474–81.

13. Maiwall R, Kumar S, Chandel SS, et al. AKI in patients with acute on chronic liver failure is different from acute decompensation of cirrhosis. Hepatol Int 2015;9(4): 627–39.

14. Allegretti AS, Ortiz G, Wenger J, et al. Prognosis of acute kidney injury and hepatorenal syndrome in patients with cirrhosis: a prospective cohort study. Int J Nephrol 2015;2015:108139.

15. Garcia-Tsao G, Parikh CR, Viola A. Acute kidney injury in cirrhosis. Hepatology 2008;48:2064–77.

16. Sherman DS, Fish DN, Teitelbaum I. Assessing renal function in cirrhotic patients: problems and pitfalls. Am J Kidney Dis 2003;41:269–78.

17. Francoz C, Prié D, Abdelrazek W, et al. Inaccuracies of creatinine and creatinine-based equations in candidates for liver transplantation with low creatinine: impact on the model for end-stage liver disease score. Liver Transpl 2010;16:1169–77.

18. Ustundag Y, Samsar U, Acikgoz S, et al. Analysis of glomerular filtration rate, serum cystatin C levels, and renal resistive index values in cirrhosis patients. Clin Chem Lab Med 2007;45:890–4.

19. Gerbes AL, Gülberg V, Bilzer M, et al. Evaluation of serum cystatin C concentration as a marker of renal function in patients with cirrhosis of the liver. Gut 2002; 50:106–10.

20. Cholongitas E, Calvaruso V, Senzolo M, et al. RIFLE classification as predictive factor of mortality in patients with cirrhosis admitted to intensive care unit. J Gastroenterol Hepatol 2009;24:1639–47.

21. Piano S, Rosi S, Maresio G, et al. Evaluation of the Acute Kidney Injury Network criteria in hospitalized patients with cirrhosis and ascites. J Hepatol 2013;59: 482–9.

22. Belcher JM, Garcia-Tsao G, Sanyal AJ, et al. Association of AKI with mortality and complications in hospitalized patients with cirrhosis. Hepatology 2013;57: 753–62.

23. Angeli P, Ginès P, Wong F, et al. Diagnosis and management of acute kidney injury in patients with cirrhosis: revised consensus recommendations of the International Club of Ascites. J Hepatol 2015;62:968–74.

24. Gines P, Schrier RW. Renal failure in cirrhosis. N Engl J Med 2009;361:1279–90.

25. Schrier RW, Shchekochikhin D, Gines P. Renal failure in cirrhosis: prerenal azotemia, hepatorenal syndrome and acute tubular necrosis. Nephrol Dial Transplant 2012;27:2625–8.

26. Arroyo V, Ginès P, Gerbes AL, et al. Definition and diagnostic criteria of refractory ascites and hepatorenal syndrome in cirrhosis. International Ascites Club. Hepatology 1996;23:164–76.

27. Salerno F, Gerbes A, Ginès P, et al. Diagnosis, prevention and treatment of hepatorenal syndrome in cirrhosis. Postgrad Med J 2008;84:662–70.

28. Ghosh S, Choudhary NS, Sharma AK, et al. Noradrenaline vs terlipressin in the treatment of type 2 hepatorenal syndrome: a randomized pilot study. Liver Int 2013;33:1187–93.

29. Fabrizi F, Aghemo A, Messa P. Hepatorenal syndrome and novel advances in its management. Kidney Blood Press Res 2013;37:588–601.

30. Velez JC, Nietert PJ. Therapeutic response to vasoconstrictors in hepatorenal syndrome parallels increase in mean arterial pressure: a pooled analysis of clinical trials. Am J Kidney Dis 2011;58:928–38.

31. Sagi SV, Mittal S, Kasturi KS, et al. Terlipressin therapy for reversal of type 1 hepatorenal syndrome: a meta-analysis of randomized controlled trials. J Gastroenterol Hepatol 2010;25:880–5.

32. Gluud LL, Christensen K, Christensen E, et al. Terlipressin for hepatorenal syndrome. Cochrane Database Syst Rev 2012;(9):CD005162.

33. Gluud LL, Christensen K, Christensen E, et al. Systematic review of randomized trials on vasoconstrictor drugs for hepatorenal syndrome. Hepatology 2010;51:576–84.

34. Ahya SN, José Soler M, Levitsky J, et al. Acid-base and potassium disorders in liver disease. Semin Nephrol 2006;26:466–70.

35. Kraut JA, Madias NE. Lactic acidosis. N Engl J Med 2014;371:2309–19.

36. Rehman HU. A woman with ketoacidosis but not diabetes. BMJ 2012;344:e1535.

37. Komatsuda A, Wakui H, Ohtani H, et al. Tubulointerstitial nephritis and renal tubular acidosis of different types are rare but important complications of primary biliary cirrhosis. Nephrol Dial Transplant 2010;25:3575–9.

38. Kraut JA, Madias NE. Treatment of acute metabolic acidosis: a pathophysiologic approach. Nat Rev Nephrol 2012;8:589–601.

39. Gonwa TA, Wadei HM. The challenges of providing renal replacement therapy in decompensated liver cirrhosis. Blood Purif 2012;33:144–8.

40. Matuszkiewicz-Rowinska J, Wieliczko M, Malyszko J. Renal replacement therapy before, during, and after orthotopic liver transplantation. Ann Transplant 2013;18:248–55.

41. Douthitt L, Bezinover D, Uemura T, et al. Perioperative use of continuous renal replacement therapy for orthotopic liver transplantation. Transplant Proc 2012;44:1314–7.

42. Parmar A, Bigam D, Meeberg G, et al. An evaluation of intraoperative renal support during liver transplantation: a matched cohort study. Blood Purif 2011;32:238–48.

43. Townsend DR, Bagshaw SM, Jacka MJ, et al. Intraoperative renal support during liver transplantation. Liver Transpl 2009;15:73–8.

44. Nadim MK, Sung RS, Davis CL, et al. Simultaneous liver-kidney transplantation summit: current state and future directions. Am J Transplant 2012;12:2901–8.

45. Parajuli S, Foley D, Djamali A, et al. Renal function and transplantation in liver disease. Transplantation 2015;99:1756–64.

46. Hmoud B, Kuo YF, Wiesner RH, et al. Outcomes of liver transplantation alone after listing for simultaneous kidney: comparison to simultaneous liver kidney transplantation. Transplantation 2015;99:823–8.

47. Martin EF, Huang J, Xiang Q, et al. Recipient survival and graft survival are not diminished by simultaneous liver-kidney transplantation: an analysis of the united network for organ sharing database. Liver Transpl 2012;18:914–29.
48. Mindikoglu AL, Raufman JP, Seliger SL, et al. Simultaneous liver-kidney versus liver transplantation alone in patients with end-stage liver disease and kidney dysfunction not on dialysis. Transplant Proc 2011;43:2669–77.
49. Francis JM, Palmer MR, Donohoe K, et al. Evaluation of native kidney recovery after simultaneous liver-kidney transplantation. Transplantation 2012;93:530–5.
50. Iglesias J, Frank E, Mehandru S, et al. Predictors of renal recovery in patients with pre-orthotopic liver transplant (OLT) renal dysfunction. BMC Nephrol 2013; 14:147.
51. Longenecker JC, Estrella MM, Segev DL, et al. Patterns of kidney function before and after orthotopic liver transplant: associations with length of hospital stay, progression to end-stage renal disease, and mortality. Transplantation 2015;99(12): 2556–64.
52. Ruebner R, Goldberg D, Abt PL, et al. Risk of end-stage renal disease among liver transplant recipients with pretransplant renal dysfunction. Am J Transplant 2012;12:2958–65.
53. Wadei HM, Geiger XJ, Cortese C, et al. Kidney allocation to liver transplant candidates with renal failure of undetermined etiology: role of percutaneous renal biopsy. Am J Transplant 2008;8:2618–26.

Respiratory Complication in Liver Disease

Vijaya S. Ramalingam, MD[a],*, Sikandar Ansari, MD[b,1], Micah Fisher, MD[c]

KEYWORDS

- Chronic liver disease • Hepatopulmonary syndrome • Hepatic hydrothorax
- Spontaneous bacterial pleuritis • Portopulmonary hypertension
- Liver transplantation

KEY POINTS

- Chronic liver disease is associated with multiple pulmonary complications.
- Hepatopulmonary syndrome, hepatic hydrothorax and portopulmonary hypertension are the most important complications with significant morbidity and mortality.
- Liver transplantation is a treatment option for eligible patients.

HEPATOPULMONARY SYNDROME

Kennedy and Knudson coined the term hepatopulmonary syndrome (HPS) in 1977. It is characterized by an oxygenation defect caused by intrapulmonary vascular dilatation (IPVD) in the setting of liver disease (**Table 1**).[1–4]

Pathophysiology

The unique pathologic feature of HPS is gross dilatation and increase in the number of pulmonary precapillary and capillary vessels to 15 to 100 μm in diameter at rest (normal range of the capillary diameter, <8–15 μm) and less commonly, pleural and pulmonary arteriovenous malformations and portopulmonary venous anastomoses.[4,5] This leads to ventilation-perfusion mismatch characterized by impaired oxygenation of venous blood caused by rapid or direct passage of mixed venous blood through the shunt into the pulmonary veins. Another mechanism is that oxygen molecules from adjacent alveoli fail to diffuse to the center of the dilated vessel to oxygenate

Disclosures: None.
[a] Division of Pulmonary & Critical Care Medicine, Department of Medicine, Medical College of Wisconsin, 9200 West Wisconsin Avenue, Milwaukee, WI 53226, USA; [b] Division of Pulmonary & Critical Care Medicine, Department of Medicine, Medical College of Wisconsin, 9200 West Wisconsin Avenue, Milwaukee, WI 53226, USA; [c] Division of Pulmonary & Critical Care Medicine, Department of Medicine, Emory Clinic 'A', 1365 Clifton Road, Northeast 4th Floor, Atlanta, GA 30322, USA
[1] Present address: 777 7th Avenue, Salt Lake City, UT 84103.
* Corresponding author.
E-mail address: vramalingam@mcw.edu

Crit Care Clin 32 (2016) 357–369
http://dx.doi.org/10.1016/j.ccc.2016.03.002
0749-0704/16/$ – see front matter © 2016 Elsevier Inc. All rights reserved.
criticalcare.theclinics.com

Table 1 Triad of HPS	
Feature	**Definition**
Liver disease	Portal hypertension with or without cirrhosis
Abnormal oxygenation	Pao_2 <80 mm Hg or A-a gradient $\geq$15 mm Hg on room air
Abnormal pulmonary vascular dilatation	Positive findings on contrast-enhanced transthoracic echocardiography or abnormal uptake in the brain (>6%) with lung perfusion scan

hemoglobin in the red blood cells in the center of venous bloodstream. This diffusion impairment is worsened by the increased cardiac output associated with liver disease because the transit time of red blood cells through the pulmonary vasculature is reduced and hence the time available for diffusion is also reduced.[1,4,6]

Multiple mechanisms have been proposed to explain IPVD. Increased pulmonary production of nitric oxide has been implicated to play a key role.[7] Studies in rats showed that there is increased activity of endothelial nitric oxide synthase and inducible nitric oxide synthase in the pulmonary microcirculation.[8,9] Enhanced hepatic production of endothelin (ET)-1 and increased expression of pulmonary vascular ET-B receptors results in nitric oxide overproduction through ET-1 mediated activation of endothelial nitric oxide synthase.[10,11] ET-1 also leads to pulmonary accumulation of monocytes, which express inducible nitric oxide synthase.[11,12] Bacterial translocation and endotoxemia also result in accumulation of macrophages in the pulmonary microcirculation.[13,14]

Nitric oxide independent mechanisms of IPVD have also been proposed: enzymatic carbon monoxide production by increased expression of heme oxygenase-1[15,16] and stimulation of calcium-activated potassium channels by endothelial-derived hyperpolarizing factor.[17] Monocytes bind to the pulmonary vasculature and produce vascular endothelial growth factor A contributing to angiogenesis, which is also identified as a major contributor to HPS.[18]

Clinical Manifestations

The estimated prevalence of HPS ranges from 5% to 32%.[4] No prospective multicenter prevalence studies have been reported to date. HPS is more common in whites than in Hispanics and African Americans, and less common in smokers.[19] It affects patients of all ages. Dyspnea on exertion, at rest, or both is the predominant presenting symptom. Platypnea and orthodeoxia (defined as dyspnea on standing and the fall in partial pressure of oxygenation in arterial blood [Pao_2] by 5% or more or by 4 mm Hg or more on standing, respectively) are present in almost 25% of patients with HPS. These are attributed to the predominance of IPVD in the lung bases, and the increase in blood flow through these regions when upright. There are no hallmark signs or symptoms of HPS. The presence of spider nevi, cyanosis, digital clubbing, and severe hypoxemia (Pao_2 <60 mm Hg) strongly suggests HPS.[20] Patients with HPS may have marked hypoxemia during sleep despite the presence of only mild to moderate daytime hypoxemia.[21] Chest radiographs may be normal or may show bibasilar nodular or reticulonodular opacities to reflect IPVD.[22] Pulmonary function tests demonstrate a consistently reduced diffusion capacity for carbon monoxide and this may not normalize after liver transplantation (LT).[23–25]

HPS can be classified as mild, moderate, severe, and very severe (**Table 2**).[4,6,20]

Table 2
Classification of HPS

Severity	A-a Gradient (mm Hg) on Room Air	Pao$_2$ (mm Hg) on Room Air
Mild	≥15	≥80
Moderate	≥15	≥60 to <80
Severe	≥15	≥50 to <60
Very severe	≥15	<50 <300 on 100% oxygen

Diagnosis

Diagnosis requires demonstration of IPVD, abnormal arterial gas exchange in the setting of underlying liver disease. More testing is required in the presence of intrinsic lung disease to attribute the degree of hypoxemia to HPS. Contrast-enhanced transthoracic echocardiography (CTTE) and lung perfusion scan are used to demonstrate IPVD and diagnose HPS. CTTE, performed by injecting agitated saline intravenously during routine transthoracic echocardiography, is the most sensitive test to detect IPVD.[8,26] The microbubbles do not pass through normal capillary diameter and are usually absorbed in the alveoli. The presence of IPVD is characterized by the delayed appearance of the microbubbles in the left atrium 3 to 6 cardiac cycles after injection as these bubbles pass through abnormally dilated pulmonary vasculature.[26]

Radionuclide lung perfusion scan with technetium-labeled macroaggregated albumin (MAA) particles is another method to demonstrate shunting. These particles, 20 to 50 μm in size, are caught in the pulmonary microvasculature of healthy individuals, whereas they shunt through the abnormal pulmonary vasculature in patients with HPS and show up in brain, kidneys, and spleen.[27,28] Degree of shunting can be calculated based on the quantitative distribution of these particles in the brain and lungs.[27] Compared with CTTE, the MAA scan is less sensitive because it cannot distinguish between intracardiac and intrapulmonary shunting.[26] However, the MAA scan may be particularly helpful in assessing the contribution of HPS to hypoxemia in patients with intrinsic lung disease with severe hypoxemia (Pao$_2$ <60 mm Hg). A prospective study in 25 patients with HPS showed that an MAA shunt greater than 6% points to HPS as the major contributor to hypoxemia.[29] MAA scan can also be used to stratify patients for postoperative mortality following LT.

Treatment

There is no effective medical therapy for the HPS. Treatment attempts with almitrine, antibiotics, garlic preparation, beta-blockers, cyclooxygenase inhibitors, systemic glucocorticoids, cyclophosphamide, inhaled nitric oxide, nitric oxide inhibitors, and somatostatin have been unsuccessful in uncontrolled trials.[4,8]

LT is the only effective treatment and can result in complete resolution of HPS or significant improvement in gas exchange. Pao$_2$ between 50 and 60 mm Hg is a firm indication for LT, whereas patients with Pao$_2$ less than 50 mm Hg should be considered on an individual basis.[1,4] A prospective study of 24 patients with cirrhosis and HPS showed a preoperative Pao$_2$ of less than 50 mm Hg alone or in combination with an MAA shunt fraction greater than 20% increased the post-LT mortality by 7.5-fold relative to patients with less severe HPS.[30] Another study showed that a pretransplantation room-air Pao$_2$ less than or equal to 44.0 mm Hg was associated with increased posttransplantation mortality.[31] Swanson and colleagues[32] showed that the 5-year survival rate of HPS without LT was only 23% compared with 76% post-LT. Recent studies also showed that post-LT mortality can be minimal in selected patients with very severe HPS.[32,33]

HEPATIC HYDROTHORAX

Hepatic hydrothorax (HH) is defined as a transudative pleural effusion, usually greater than 500 mL in patients with portal hypertension in the absence of underlying primary cardiac, pulmonary, or pleural diseases.

Pathophysiology

Portal hypertension is essential in the development of ascites and HH. The passage of ascitic fluid from the peritoneal cavity to the pleural space via small diaphragmatic defects called pleuroperitoneal communications or blebs is considered the key mechanism. These communications are predominantly seen on the right hemidiaphragm and are usually less than 1 cm in size.[8] The right-sided predominance is caused by the close anatomic relationship of bare areas of the liver with the diaphragm. Also, the left hemidiaphram is thicker and more muscular than the right. The increasing abdominal pressure caused by ascites and the diaphragmatic thinning caused by malnutrition in patients with cirrhosis enlarge these defects. The negative intrathoracic pressure during inspiration also contributes to the one-way flow from peritoneal cavity to the pleural space.

Clinical Manifestation

HH is seen in approximately 5% to 10% of patients with cirrhosis.[34,35] In a study of 1038 patients with cirrhosis, HH was seen in 49 patients (4.72%).[36] Another study showed pleural effusion in 15% of patients with cirrhosis but only 6.5% had enough fluid to perform a thoracentesis.[37]

HH should always be suspected in a patient with cirrhosis with pleural effusion, typically right-sided effusion. Depending on the amount of pleural effusion, rapidity of accumulation, and underlying pulmonary disease, patients present with cough, dyspnea, chest discomfort, or acute respiratory failure.

Diagnosis

Ascites is not required for diagnosis of HH. Up to 20% patients with HH have no clinically significant ascites. Thoracoabdominal scintigraphy with intraperitoneal administration of Tc99 m colloid and detection of colloid in the pleural space, even in the absence of underlying ascites, has confirmed the existence of pleuroperitoneal communications.[38] However, this is rarely used in the clinical practice.

Chest radiography is used to confirm the presence of a pleural effusion. Although most effusions are unilateral and right-sided, a small subset of patients may have bilateral and/or left-sided effusions. A study of 1038 patients with cirrhosis showed that HH was right-sided in 34 (69.4%), bilateral in nine (18.4%), and left-sided in six (12.2%).[36] In a retrospective study of 60 patients with cirrhosis with pleural effusions, uncomplicated HH was found in 42 patients (70%), whereas the rest of the patients were found to have infected HH and causes other than liver disease. A total of 80% of right-sided effusions were uncomplicated, whereas only 35% of left-sided effusions were uncomplicated.[39] Hence the presence of left-sided pleural effusion should not be assumed to be uncomplicated.

Pleural fluid analysis is mandatory to confirm HH and rule out other causes of pleural effusion, such as infection or cancer. The characteristics of uncomplicated HH are listed in **Box 1**.[36,40]

Box 1
Laboratory characteristics of HH

Uncomplicated

- Polymorphonuclear cell count <250
- Total protein concentration <2.5 g/dL
- Pleural fluid total protein/serum total protein ratio <0.5
- Pleural fluid lactate dehydrogenase/serum lactate dehydrogenase <0.6
- Serum to pleural fluid albumin gradient >1.1 g/dL
- pH 7.4 to 7.55
- Pleural fluid/serum bilirubin ratio <0.6
- Glucose level similar to that of serum

Spontaneous bacterial pleuritis

- Positive pleural fluid culture and a polymorphonuclear cell >250 OR
- Negative pleural fluid culture and a polymorphonuclear cell >500 AND
- Absence of pneumonia or contiguous infection on chest imaging

---

Depending on the clinical circumstances, chest computed tomography to exclude mediastinal, pulmonary, and pleural lesions, echocardiography to evaluate for heart failure, or abdominal ultrasound with Doppler to assess the patency of portal and hepatic veins may also be needed.

Treatment

Patients with HH should be evaluated for LT because it heralds decompensating liver disease. The goals of treatment are to provide symptomatic relief and prevent pulmonary complications and infections until LT is performed.

Similar to management of ascites, sodium restriction and diuretics are effective in controlling HH. However 20% of patients may develop refractory HH because fluid mobilization from the pleural cavity may be slower than from the peritoneal cavity.[41]

In patients with refractory HH, therapeutic thoracentesis is well tolerated and effective in relieving dyspnea, but is associated with an increased risk of infection, bleeding, pneumothorax, and protein loss. It is suggested that if a patient requires therapeutic thoracentesis every 2 to 3 weeks despite maximal sodium restriction and adequate diuretics, alternative treatments should be considered because of increased complication rates.[35–40] Thoracenteses are often limited to draining no more than 1 to 2 L because of the risk of re-expansion pulmonary edema. But a study of 185 patients undergoing large-volume thoracentesis showed that re-expansion pulmonary edema is rare and independent of the volume of fluid removed, pleural pressures, and pleural elastance. Large effusions can be drained safely if no chest discomfort develops or end-expiratory pleural pressure remains below −20 cm H_2O.[42]

Transjugular intrahepatic portosystemic shunt is effective for refractory hydrothorax and should be considered in selected patients with a Child-Pugh score less than 10, age less than 60 years, and without any evidence of hepatic encephalopathy.[43] Video-assisted thoracoscopic surgery with pleurodesis is reserved as a palliative measure in selected patients where medical therapy and transjugular intrahepatic portosystemic shunt have failed. Fluid control with pleurodesis is inferior to transjugular intrahepatic portosystemic shunt because of rapid reaccumulation of pleural fluid.

Chest tube placement is contraindicated in the absence of empyema because of the risk of fluid depletion, protein loss, infection caused by poor wound healing, fluid depletion, and renal failure.[44]

SPONTANEOUS BACTERIAL PLEURITIS

Spontaneous bacterial pleuritis (SBPL) is defined as infected HH in the absence of pneumonia. Although spontaneous bacterial empyema is more commonly used, the presence of pus in the pleural space is not required for its diagnosis. The incidence of SBPL is similar to spontaneous bacterial peritonitis (SBP), which is reported between 15% and 20% in hospitalized patients with cirrhosis with ascites. In a study of 3390 patients with cirrhosis, SBPL was seen in 2.4% of patients with cirrhosis and 16% of patients with cirrhosis with hydrothorax.[44] Other studies also showed similar incidence for SBPL: 2% in patients with cirrhosis and 13% in patients with cirrhosis with hydrothorax.[37,39,45]

In contrary to the popular belief that the flow of infected peritoneal fluid to the pleural space causes SBPL, studies demonstrated that SBPL was not associated with SBP in more than 40% patients and hence a thoracentesis should be performed when paracentesis is negative and infection is suspected.[43,44] Enteric microorganisms entering the pleural space by spontaneous bacteremia is also postulated.[35,37] The microorganisms most commonly involved are Enterobacteriaceae (Escherichia coli and Klebsiella pneumonia), Streptococcus species, and Enterococcus species and these are also the most common bacterial causes of SBP.

A high level of suspicion is required because patients with SBPL may present with fever, pleuritic chest pain, worsening mental status, or renal function. The diagnosis of SBPL needs a positive pleural fluid culture and a polymorphonuclear cell greater than 250 cells/mm^3 or a negative pleural fluid culture and a polymorphonuclear cell greater than 500 cells/mm^3 in the absence of pneumonia or contiguous infection on chest imaging.[46,47] Patients with advanced liver disease, higher Child-Pugh score, low pleural fluid total protein (<1 mg/dL), and C3 levels are at increased risk of developing SBPL.[37,39,48]

Treatment

Treatment of SBPL is typically with third-generation cephalosporins. Prophylactic antibiotic therapy should be initiated after an episode of SBPL. Xiol and colleagues[45] showed that the mortality associated with SBPL was 20%.[44] Unlike in SBP, the use of albumin to prevent hepatorenal syndrome has not been studied in patients with SBPL. Similar to patients with HH, chest tube placement is contraindicated in the absence of empyema.[44,49]

PORTOPULMONARY HYPERTENSION

Portopulmonary hypertension (POPH) is the elevation of pulmonary artery pressure caused by increased pulmonary vascular resistance (PVR) in the setting of portal hypertension.[50] It is characterized by mean pulmonary artery pressure (mPAP) of greater than 25 mm Hg, pulmonary artery occlusion pressure of less than 15 mm Hg, and PVR of greater than 240 dyn/s/cm^{-5} in the presence of portal hypertension, with or without advanced liver disease.[20] It was first reported by Mantz and Craige in 1951.[51] They described a 53-year-old woman with portal vein thrombosis with spontaneous portocaval shunt and an enlarged pulmonary artery. Autopsy revealed intimal thickening of medium and large pulmonary arteries and endothelial proliferation of terminal pulmonary arterioles.

Epidemiology

A large autopsy study showed that pulmonary hypertension (PH) was five times more likely in patients with cirrhosis than those without liver disease. In a study of 1235 patients, 66 patients (5.3%) were found to have POPH.[52] In another study of 507 patients with portal hypertension, 2% were found to have POPH.[53] POPH was diagnosed in 5.3% of the cases (174 of 3525) in the REVEAL registry (Registry to Evaluate Early and Long-term Pulmonary Arterial Hypertension Disease Management).[54]

Clinical Manifestations

The symptoms and signs of POPH are similar to those in other types of pulmonary arterial hypertension and depend on the severity of POPH. Exertional dyspnea is the most common presenting symptom in more than 80% of patients.[55] As the disease progresses, patients can present with fatigue, chest pain, and dyspnea at rest. Patients with mild POPH may only show stigmata of liver disease, such as jaundice, palmar erythema, ascites, and lower extremity swelling. A loud pulmonary component of the second heart sound, a left parasternal heave, jugular venous distention, along with other signs of right heart failure may be noticed as the disease progresses.[44,56,57]

Pathogenesis

Several mechanisms have been proposed including genetic predisposition, pulmonary vascular wall stress, and increased vasoactive metabolites. The pathogenesis of POPH is unclear and is likely multifactorial.

Increased splanchnic circulation and extensive portosystemic shunts associated with portal hypertension allows the blood from gastrointestinal tract to bypass the liver and its normal metabolic functions. This exposes the pulmonary vasculature to potent vasoactive substances, such as ET-1, interleukin-1 and -6, vasoactive intestinal peptide, glucagon, serotonin, thromboxane, bacteria, and endotoxins.[58] Liver specimens obtained from 62 patients with cirrhosis at the time of LT showed higher levels of ET-1 compared with control subjects. ET-1, a potent systemic and pulmonary vasoconstrictor, also aggravates portal hypertension by increasing the hepatic stellate cell contraction and sinusoidal tone. Studies have shown elevated systemic and splanchnic ET-1 levels in patients with cirrhosis and POPH compared with patients with cirrhosis without POPH. Prostacyclin, a potent vasodilator and inhibitor of platelet adhesion and cell growth, is also decreased in patients with POPH because of deficiency of endothelial prostacyclin synthase in lung parenchyma. The role of ET-1 and prostacyclin in POPH is also supported by the therapeutic role of ET-1 antagonists and prostacyclin analogues.[59–62]

Peripheral vascular resistance is reduced in patients with liver disease. To compensate for this, cardiac output is increased to increase the pulmonary blood flow. This persistent circulatory overload may potentially cause pulmonary vascular wall stress. Genetic variation in estrogen signaling, oxidative stress, and cell growth/apoptosis regulator genes is also associated with increased risk of POPH.[63] These factors and possibly other yet undiscovered mechanisms cause characteristic pulmonary vascular pathology indistinguishable from other phenotypes of pulmonary arterial hypertension, which includes intimal fibrosis, endothelial and smooth muscle cell proliferation, in situ thrombosis, and plexogenic arteriopathy.[64,65]

Diagnosis

As with other forms of PH, transthoracic echocardiography is an important screening tool for POPH. A right ventricular (RV) systolic pressure of 30 to 50 mm Hg is generally considered suspicious for underlying PH. With structural signs of RV failure on the echocardiogram (D-shaped septum, right atrial or RV dilatation, and so forth) values of the RV systolic pressure as low as 30 mm Hg should also be considered as a sign of PH. Studies have shown that an RV systolic pressure cutoff of 38 mm Hg had an acceptable sensitivity and a specificity of 82%, along with a PPV of 22%. If RV dilatation was added to this variable, then the sensitivity remained acceptable, and the specificity and PPV improved to 92% and 41%, respectively.[66,67]

A right heart catheterization is extremely important in differentiating POPH from hyper dynamic state because of liver disease and volume overload (**Table 3**). When the mPAP is higher than 25 mm Hg, with a pulmonary capillary wedge pressure (PCWP) lower than 15 mm Hg and PVR higher than 240 dyn/s/cm^{-5}, then in the right clinical setting the diagnosis of POPH can be made. When the mPAP is higher than 25 mm Hg, with a PCWP lower than 15 mm Hg and PVR lower than 240 dyn/s/cm^{-5}, the elevated mPAP is related to the hyperdynamic state and not caused by pulmonary arterial remodeling typical in POPH and other patients with PAH.[20,67,68]

Treatment

The goals of therapy in this patient population include symptomatic relief, improvement in exercise capacity, and facilitate LT in a select group of patients.

Supplemental oxygen is universally used to prevent hypoxia, and diuretics are used to manage the overall volume status and also off-load a dilated RV.[68] Volume status management in these patients is challenging because they also have decreased venous return and are prone to prerenal azotemia. Calcium channel blockers are reserved for a small group of patients with idiopathic pulmonary arterial hypertension who have a positive vasoreactivity test. However, they are contraindicated in POPH because they may cause splanchnic vasodilation and worsen portal hypertension.[69] Beta-blockers are used as prophylaxis for variceal hemorrhage, but some clinicians avoid them because of a negative chronotropic and inotropic affect, which may make the PH worse.[70]

Identifying the correct patient for PH-specific therapy is extremely important (see **Table 3**). Patients with an elevated mPAP caused by hyperdynamic state related to liver disease should not be treated with PH-specific therapy. Patients with an elevated mPAP, normal PCWP and an elevated PVR (>240 dyn/s/cm^{-5}) are candidates for POPH-specific therapies.

Pulmonary vasodilators can be used as a definitive therapy to treat the POPH, or also as a bridge to transplantation. Prostanoids, ET receptor antagonists, and

Table 3
Hemodynamic patterns on right heart catheterization in patients with advanced liver disease

Hemodynamic Pattern	Mean Pulmonary Artery Pressure	Pulmonary Vascular Resistance	Pulmonary Artery Occlusion Pressure	Cardiac Output
Hyperdynamic circulation	Increased	Normal	Normal	Increased
Pulmonary venous hypertension	Increased	Normal or mildly increased	Increased	Increased
Portopulmonary hypertension	Increased	Increased	Normal	Initially increased and decreases as pulmonary vascular resistance rises

phosphodiesterase inhibitors have all showed good outcomes.[71–75] Patients require close monitoring of liver function tests if they are treated with endothelin receptor antagonists, especially bosentan. These agents along with newer ones approved to treat PH are available to be used alone or in combination and should be chosen based on the individual's disease severity and ability to tolerate side effects, with the intravenous prostanoids reserved for the more severe disease.

Patients who are candidates for liver transplant are placed on the transplant list and also scored against the MELD scoring system with the addition of the MELD exception point for POPH. The system is as follows.[76]

1. Moderate to severe POPH diagnosis by right heart catheterization (RHC)
   a. mPAP $\geq$35 mm Hg
   b. PVR >400 dyn/s/cm^{-5}
   c. pulmonary artery occlusion pressure $\leq$15 mm Hg
2. Improvement with PAH-specific therapies by
   a. mPAP <35 mm Hg or,
   b. PVR <400 dyn/s/cm^{-5} regardless of mPAP and,
   c. Satisfactory RV function by transthoracic echocardiography (eg, improvement in RV dilation and function)
3. MELD exceptions updated (additional 10% MELD points) every 3 months
   a. Give additional MELD exception if RHC data satisfy criteria #2.

The goal of this exception is to facilitate LT in patients with POPH while the hemodynamics is still favorable. An mPAP greater than 45 mm Hg and PVR greater than 400 dyn/s/cm−5 are absolute contraindications for LT. Even with an mPAP greater than 35 mm Hg, the peritransplant mortality can be up to 50%.[77] Pulmonary vasodilators should be used to bring the mPAP lower than 45 mm Hg, ideally even lower, and to bring the PVR lower than 250 dyn/s/cm^{-5} before LT is attempted.

All patients with POPH should be referred to an experienced high-volume center for pulmonary vasodilator therapy, and LT should be undertaken where invasive, intraoperative cardiac monitoring is possible. In experienced centers, pretransplant pulmonary vasodilator therapy followed by LT shows survival outcomes similar to all LT for all indications.[78]

SUMMARY

There are multiple pulmonary complications associated with chronic liver disease. Patients with cirrhosis who complain of dyspnea should be evaluated for the diseases discussed here. HPS is the most common one and LT is the only effective treatment that can result in complete resolution of HPS or significant improvement in gas exchange. Patients with HH should also be evaluated for LT because it heralds decompensating liver disease. Patients with moderate POPH and good response to medical therapy may be considered for LT, whereas the presence of severe POPH may preclude LT.

REFERENCES

1. Singh C, Sager JS. Pulmonary complications of cirrhosis. Med Clin North Am 2009;93(4):871–83.
2. Kung HC, Hoyert DL, Xu J, et al. Deaths: final data for 2005. Natl Vital Stat Rep 2008;56(10):1–120.
3. Kennedy TC, Knudson RJ. Exercise-aggravated hypoxemia and orthodeoxia in cirrhosis. Chest 1977;72(3):305–9.

4. Rodríguez-Roisin R, Krowka MJ. Hepatopulmonary syndrome: a liver-induced lung vascular disorder. N Engl J Med 2008;358(22):2378–87.
5. Berthelot P, Walker JG, Sherlock S, et al. Arterial changes in the lungs in cirrhosis of the liver–lung spider nevi. N Engl J Med 1966;274(6):291–8.
6. Rodriguez-Roisin R, Roca J, Agusti AG, et al. Gas exchange and pulmonary vascular reactivity in patients with liver cirrhosis. Am Rev Respir Dis 1987; 135(5):1085–92.
7. Cremona G, Higenbottam TW, Mayoral V, et al. Elevated exhaled nitric oxide in patients with hepatopulmonary syndrome. Eur Respir J 1995;8(11):1883–5.
8. Machicao VI, Balakrishnan M, Fallon MB. Pulmonary complications in chronic liver disease. Hepatology 2014;59(4):1627–37.
9. Fallon MB, Abrams GA, Luo B, et al. The role of endothelial nitric oxide synthase in the pathogenesis of a rat model of hepatopulmonary syndrome. Gastroenterology 1997;113(2):606–14.
10. Fallon MB, Abrams GA, McGrath JW, et al. Common bile duct ligation in the rat: a model of intrapulmonary vasodilatation and hepatopulmonary syndrome. Am J Physiol 1997;272(4 Pt 1):G779–84.
11. Tang L, Luo B, Patel RP, et al. Modulation of pulmonary endothelial endothelin B receptor expression and signaling: implications for experimental hepatopulmonary syndrome. Am J Physiol Lung Cell Mol Physiol 2007;292(6):L1467–72.
12. Ling Y, Zhang J, Luo B, et al. The role of endothelin-1 and the endothelin B receptor in the pathogenesis of hepatopulmonary syndrome in the rat. Hepatology 2004;39(6):1593–602.
13. Rabiller A, Nunes H, Lebrec D, et al. Prevention of gram-negative translocation reduces the severity of hepatopulmonary syndrome. Am J Respir Crit Care Med 2002;166(4):514–7.
14. Thenappan T, Goel A, Marsboom G, et al. A central role for CD68(+) macrophages in hepatopulmonary syndrome. Reversal by macrophage depletion. Am J Respir Crit Care Med 2011;183(8):1080–91.
15. Carter EP, Hartsfield CL, Miyazono M, et al. Regulation of heme oxygenase-1 by nitric oxide during hepatopulmonary syndrome. Am J Physiol Lung Cell Mol Physiol 2002;283(2):L346–53.
16. Zhang J, Ling Y, Luo B, et al. Analysis of pulmonary heme oxygenase-1 and nitric oxide synthase alterations in experimental hepatopulmonary syndrome. Gastroenterology 2003;125(5):1441–51.
17. Carter EP, Sato K, Morio Y, et al. Inhibition of K(Ca) channels restores blunted hypoxic pulmonary vasoconstriction in rats with cirrhosis. Am J Physiol Lung Cell Mol Physiol 2000;279(5):L903–10.
18. Zhang J, Luo B, Tang L, et al. Pulmonary angiogenesis in a rat model of hepatopulmonary syndrome. Gastroenterology 2009;136(3):1070–80.
19. Fallon MB, Krowka MJ, Brown RS, et al, Pulmonary Vascular Complications of Liver Disease Study Group. Impact of hepatopulmonary syndrome on quality of life and survival in liver transplant candidates. Gastroenterology 2008;135(4): 1168–75.
20. Rodríguez-Roisin R, Krowka MJ, Hervé P, et al, ERS Task Force Pulmonary-Hepatic Vascular Disorders (PHD) Scientific Committee. Pulmonary-Hepatic vascular Disorders (PHD). Eur Respir J 2004;24(5):861–80.
21. Palma DT, Philips GM, Arguedas MR, et al. Oxygen desaturation during sleep in hepatopulmonary syndrome. Hepatology 2008;47(4):1257–63.
22. McAdams HP, Erasmus J, Crockett R, et al. The hepatopulmonary syndrome: radiologic findings in 10 patients. AJR Am J Roentgenol 1996;166(6):1379–85.

23. Martínez GP, Barberà JA, Visa J, et al. Hepatopulmonary syndrome in candidates for liver transplantation. J Hepatol 2001;34(5):651–7.

24. Battaglia SE, Pretto JJ, Irving LB, et al. Resolution of gas exchange abnormalities and intrapulmonary shunting following liver transplantation. Hepatology 1997; 25(5):1228–32.

25. Martínez-Palli G, Gómez FP, Barberà JA, et al. Sustained low diffusing capacity in hepatopulmonary syndrome after liver transplantation. World J Gastroenterol 2006;12(36):5878–83.

26. Abrams GA, Jaffe CC, Hoffer PB, et al. Diagnostic utility of contrast echocardiography and lung perfusion scan in patients with hepatopulmonary syndrome. Gastroenterology 1995;109(4):1283–8.

27. Wolfe JD, Tashkin DP, Holly FE, et al. Hypoxemia of cirrhosis: detection of abnormal small pulmonary vascular channels by a quantitative radionuclide method. Am J Med 1977;63(5):746–54.

28. Abrams GA, Nanda NC, Dubovsky EV, et al. Use of macroaggregated albumin lung perfusion scan to diagnose hepatopulmonary syndrome: a new approach. Gastroenterology 1998;114(2):305–10.

29. Krowka MJ, Wiseman GA, Burnett OL, et al. Hepatopulmonary syndrome: a prospective study of relationships between severity of liver disease, PaO(2) response to 100% oxygen, and brain uptake after (99m)Tc MAA lung scanning. Chest 2000;118(3):615–24.

30. Arguedas MR, Abrams GA, Krowka MJ, et al. Prospective evaluation of outcomes and predictors of mortality in patients with hepatopulmonary syndrome undergoing liver transplantation. Hepatology 2003;37(1):192–7.

31. Goldberg DS, Krok K, Batra S, et al. Impact of the hepatopulmonary syndrome MELD exception policy on outcomes of patients after liver transplantation: an analysis of the UNOS database. Gastroenterology 2014;146(5):1256–65.

32. Swanson KL, Wiesner RH, Krowka MJ. Natural history of hepatopulmonary syndrome: impact of liver transplantation. Hepatology 2005;41(5):1122–9.

33. Gupta S, Castel H, Rao RV, et al. Improved survival after liver transplantation in patients with hepatopulmonary syndrome. Am J Transplant 2010;10(2):354–63.

34. Huang TW, Cheng YL, Chang H, et al. Education and imaging. Hepatobiliary and pancreatic: hepatic hydrothorax. J Gastroenterol Hepatol 2007;22(6):956.

35. Norvell JP, Spivey JR. Hepatic hydrothorax. Clin Liver Dis 2014;18(2):439–49.

36. Malagari K, Nikita A, Alexopoulou E, et al. Cirrhosis-related intrathoracic disease. Imaging features in 1038 patients. Hepatogastroenterology 2005;52(62):558–62.

37. Chen TA, Lo GH, Lai KH. Risk factors for spontaneous bacterial empyema in cirrhotic patients with hydrothorax. J Chin Med Assoc 2003;66(10):579–86.

38. Benet A, Vidal F, Toda R, et al. Diagnosis of hepatic hydrothorax in the absence of ascites by intraperitoneal injection of 99m-Tc-Fluor colloid. Postgrad Med J 1992; 68(796):153.

39. Xiol X, Castellote J, Cortes-Beut R, et al. Usefulness and complications of thoracentesis in cirrhotic patients. Am J Med 2001;111(1):67–9.

40. Krok KL, Cárdenas A. Hepatic hydrothorax. Semin Respir Crit Care Med 2012; 33(1):3–10.

41. Siegerstetter V, Deibert P, Ochs A, et al. Treatment of refractory hepatic hydrothorax with transjugular intrahepatic portosystemic shunt: long-term results in 40 patients. Eur J Gastroenterol Hepatol 2001;13(5):529–34.

42. Feller-Kopman D, Berkowitz D, Boiselle P, et al. Large-volume thoracentesis and the risk of reexpansion pulmonary edema. Ann Thorac Surg 2007;84(5):1656–61.

43. Wilputte JY, Goffette P, Zech F, et al. The outcome after transjugular intrahepatic portosystemic shunt (TIPS) for hepatic hydrothorax is closely related to liver dysfunction: a long-term study in 28 patients. Acta Gastroenterol Belg 2007; 70(1):6–10.

44. Chen CH, Shih CM, Chou JW, et al. Outcome predictors of cirrhotic patients with spontaneous bacterial empyema. Liver Int 2011;31(3):417–24.

45. Xiol X, Castellví JM, Guardiola J, et al. Spontaneous bacterial empyema in cirrhotic patients: a prospective study. Hepatology 1996;23(4):719–23.

46. Gurung P, Goldblatt M, Huggins JT, et al. Pleural fluid analysis and radiographic, sonographic, and echocardiographic characteristics of hepatic hydrothorax. Chest 2011;140(2):448–53.

47. Tu CY, Chen CH. Spontaneous bacterial empyema. Curr Opin Pulm Med 2012; 18(4):355–8.

48. Sese E, Xiol X, Castellote J, et al. Low complement levels and opsonic activity in hepatic hydrothorax: its relationship with spontaneous bacterial empyema. J Clin Gastroenterol 2003;36(1):75–7.

49. Runyon BA, Greenblatt M, Ming RH. Hepatic hydrothorax is a relative contraindication to chest tube insertion. Am J Gastroenterol 1986;81(7):566–7.

50. Simonneau G, Gatzoulis MA, Adatia I, et al. Updated clinical classification of pulmonary hypertension. J Am Coll Cardiol 2013;62(25 Suppl):D34–41.

51. Mantz FA Jr, Craige E. Portal axis thrombosis with spontaneous portacaval shunt and resultant cor pulmonale. AMA Arch Pathol 1951;52:91–7.

52. Krowka MJ, Swanson KL, Frantz RP, et al. Portopulmonary hypertension: results from a 10-year screening algorithm. Hepatology 2006;44(6):1502–10.

53. Hadengue A, Benhayoun MK, Lebrec D, et al. Pulmonary hypertension complicating portal hypertension: prevalence and relation to splanchnic hemodynamics. Gastroenterology 1991;100(2):520–8.

54. Krowka MJ, Miller DP, Barst RJ, et al. Portopulmonary hypertension: a report from the US-based REVEAL Registry. Chest 2012;141(4):906–15.

55. Medarov BI, Chopra A, Judson MA. Clinical aspects of portopulmonary hypertension. Respir Med 2014;108(7):943–54.

56. Robalino BD, Moodie DS. Association between primary pulmonary hypertension and portal hypertension: analysis of its pathophysiology and clinical, laboratory and hemodynamic manifestations. J Am Coll Cardiol 1991;17(2):492–8.

57. Pilatis ND, Jacobs LE, Rerkpattanapipat P, et al. Clinical predictors of pulmonary hypertension in patients undergoing liver transplant evaluation. Liver Transpl 2000;6(1):85–91.

58. Herve P, Launay JM, Scrobohaci ML, et al. Increased plasma serotonin levels in primary pulmonary hypertension. Am J Med 1995;99:249–54.

59. Benjaminov FS, Prentice M, Sniderman KW, et al. Portopulmonary hypertension in decompensated liver cirrhosis and refractory ascites. Gut 2003;52:1355–62.

60. Kamath PS, Carpenter HA, Lloyd RV, et al. Hepatic localization of endothelin-1 in patients with idiopathic portal hypertension and cirrhosis of the liver. Liver Transpl 2000;6:596–602.

61. Neuhofer W, Gulberg V, Gerbes AL. Endothelin and endothelin receptor antagonism in portopulmonary hypertension. Eur J Clin Invest 2006;36(Suppl 3):54–61.

62. Tuder RM, Cool CD, Geraci MW, et al. Prostacyclin synthase expression is decreased in lungs from patients with severe pulmonary hypertension. Am J Respir Crit Care Med 1999;159:1925–32.

63. Roberts KE, Fallon MB, Krowka MJ, et al. Genetic risk factors for portopulmonary hypertension in patients with advanced liver disease. Am J Respir Crit Care Med 2009;179:835–42.
64. Edwards BS, Weir EK, Edwards WD, et al. Coexistent pulmonary and portal hypertension: morphologic and clinical features. J Am Coll Cardiol 1987;10:1233–8.
65. Krowka MJ, Edwards WD. A spectrum of pulmonary vascular pathology in portopulmonary hypertension. Liver Transpl 2000;6:241–2.
66. Raevens S, Colle IO, Reyntjens K, et al. Echocardiography for the detection of portopulmonary hypertension in liver transplantation candidates: analysis of different cut-off values. Liver Transpl 2013;19:602–10.
67. Porres-Aguilar M, Duarte-Rojo A, Krowka MJ. Transthoracic echocardiography screening for the detection of portopulmonary hypertension: work in progress. Liver Transpl 2013;19:573–4.
68. Porres-Aguilar M, Altamirano JT, Torre-Delgadillo A, et al. Portopulmonary hypertension and hepatopulmonary syndrome: a clinician-oriented overview. Eur Respir Rev 2012;21:223–33.
69. Ota K, Shijo H, Kokawa H, et al. Effects of nifedipine on hepatic venous pressure gradient and portal vein flow in patient with cirrhosis. J Gastroenterol Hepatol 1995;10:198–204.
70. Provencher S, Herve P, Jais X, et al. Deleterious effects of beta-blockers on exercise capacity and hemodynamics in patients with portopulmonary hypertension. Gastroenterology 2006;130:120–6.
71. Krowka MJ, Frantz RP, McGoon MD, et al. Improvement in pulmonary hemodynamics during intravenous epoprostenol: a study of 15 patients with moderate and severe portopulmonary hypertension. Hepatology 1999;30:641–8.
72. Fix OK, Bass NM, De Marco T, et al. Long-term follow up in portopulmonary hypertension: effect of treatment with epoprostenol. Liver Transpl 2007;13:875–85.
73. Sussman N, Kaza V, Barshes N, et al. Successful liver transplantation following medical management of portopulmonary hypertension: a single center series. Am J Transplant 2006;6:2177–82.
74. Hoeper MM, Halank M, Marx C, et al. Bosentan therapy for portopulmonary hypertension. Eur Respir J 2005;25:502–8.
75. Reichenberger F, Voswinckel R, Steveling E, et al. Sildenafil treatment for portopulmonary hypertension. Eur Respir J 2006;28:563–7.
76. Krowka MJ, Fallon MB, Mulligan DC, et al. Model for endstage liver disease (MELD) exception for portopulmonary hypertension. Liver Transpl 2006; 12(Suppl 3):S114–6.
77. Krowka MJ, Mandell SM, Ramsay MA, et al. Hepatopulmonary syndrome and portopulmonary hypertension: a report from the multicenter liver transplant database. Liver Transpl 2004;10:174–82.
78. Ashfaq M, Chinnakotla S, Rogers L, et al. The impact of treatment of portopulmonary hypertension on survival following liver transplantation. Am J Transplant 2007;7:1258–64.

Gastrointestinal Issues in Liver Disease

Jody C. Olson, MD[a],*, Kia Saeian, MD, MSc Epi[b]

KEYWORDS

- Liver disease • Gastrointestinal issues • Variceal hemorrhage • Gastric varices
- Portal hypertensive gastropathy • Cirrhosis

KEY POINTS

- Gastrointestinal (GI) complications are frequent in cirrhotic patients admitted to the intensive care unit.
- Bleeding from gastric or esophageal varices results in significant morbidity and mortality in cirrhotic patients.
- Nonvariceal GI blood loss is also frequently seen in cirrhosis and may be difficult to manage; this includes portal hypertensive gastropathy and gastric vascular ectasia.
- Cirrhotic patients frequently have significant malnutrition prompting the need for early nutritional support in this patient population.

INTRODUCTION

The frequency of gastrointestinal (GI) complications of advanced liver disease mirrors the progression of fibrosis and portal hypertension, which occurs during the natural history of cirrhosis. Remembering that pressure is directly proportional to resistance and flow ($P \propto Resistance \times Flow$), where P is pressure, one can examine how portal venous pressures may be increased in cirrhosis via a complex interplay of physical and biochemical alterations. Progressive deposition of extracellular matrix leads to architectural disruption of normal hepatic blood flow and, thus, contributes to portal hypertension via increased resistance. In addition to the structural component of increased resistance, biochemical abnormalities also contribute to increasing portal pressures seen in advanced liver disease. Since the first study demonstrating a reversible element of intrahepatic vascular resistance could be induced by vasodilators in 1985,[1] our understanding of the mechanisms responsible for this phenomenon has continued to evolve. The free radical nitric oxide (NO) is an important mediator of vascular resistance in biological systems. Rat models of portal hypertension

[a] The University of Kansas, 3901 Rainbow Boulevard, Kansas City, KS 66160, USA; [b] Medical College of Wisconsin, 9200 West Wisconsin Avenue, Milwaukee, WI 53226, USA
* Corresponding author.
E-mail address: jolson2@kumc.edu

Crit Care Clin 32 (2016) 371–384
http://dx.doi.org/10.1016/j.ccc.2016.03.007
0749-0704/16/$ – see front matter © 2016 Elsevier Inc. All rights reserved.

demonstrate NO as mediator in the development of portal hypertension via 2 important mechanisms influencing both resistance and flow. First, endothelial dysfunction in cirrhosis results in a decrease in NO production within the liver, which results in an increase in intrahepatic vascular resistance.[2,3] Second, in contrast to the decreased NO production within the liver, NO production is increased within the splanchnic vasculature leading to increases in portal blood flow further exacerbating portal hypertension.[4,5] This reversible component provides a potential target for therapeutic intervention with vasoactive agents.

GASTROINTESTINAL BLEEDING
Esophageal Varices

Esophageal varices are present in approximately 50% of cirrhotic patients at the time cirrhosis is diagnosed.[6] Esophageal varices develop at a rate of 8% per year, and those with small varices may progress to large varices at a rate of approximately 8% to 10% per year.[7,8] As described earlier, the risk of bleeding from gastroesophageal varices (GOV) is proportional to the degree of portal hypertension. Perhaps the most widely accepted tool to assess portal hypertension is the hepatic venous pressure gradient (HVPG), which provides an indirect measure of portal pressures. The HVPG is the difference obtained by directly measuring the free hepatic venous pressure (FHVP) and by obtaining a wedged hepatic venous pressure (WHVP) via an occlusion balloon (HVPG = WHVP − FHVP).[9] The normal HVPG is between 3 and 5 mm Hg with an HVPG of 10 mm Hg or greater being significantly associated with the presence of GOV and an HVPG of greater than 12 mm Hg typically associated with a risk of hemorrhage.[8] Although the HVPG has proven extremely valuable in our understanding of the pathophysiology of portal hypertension, its practical application at the bedside can be cumbersome and has limitations leading to a lack of routine application particularly in the United States.

Rupture of GOV is one of the most lethal complications of advanced portal hypertension. Rupture of portosystemic varices may result in death directly from massive exsanguination but may also contribute to death from propagation of acute-on-chronic liver failure or progressive hepatic decompensation. Mortality rates associated with variceal hemorrhage, which were traditionally reported to be as high as 50%, have more recently decreased to 33.5%, a decrease attributed to improvements in treatment modalities and critical care management.[10]

Management of Acute Esophageal Hemorrhage

Patients presenting with acute esophageal variceal hemorrhage should be admitted to an intensive care setting with adherence to basic life support procedures including an initial focus on airway management and hemodynamic support. For actively bleeding patients with concomitant hepatic encephalopathy who are being prepared to undergo endoscopy, the preferred method for airway control is endotracheal intubation. Resuscitation targets for hemoglobin were established in a randomized controlled trial demonstrating when a restrictive transfusion threshold of 7 g/dL is used compared with a more liberal strategy of 9 g/dL; patients with Childs A or B disease had significantly better survival (hazard ratio, 0.30; 95% confidence interval [CI] 0.11–0.85) and fewer adverse events ($P = .02$).[11]

Initial directed therapies for treatment of bleeding esophageal varices include prompt initiation of vasoactive agents and antibiotics followed by endoscopic therapy, which may include sclerotherapy or, preferably, endoscopic band ligation (EVL) (**Fig. 1**). Once esophageal variceal hemorrhage is suspected, early administration of

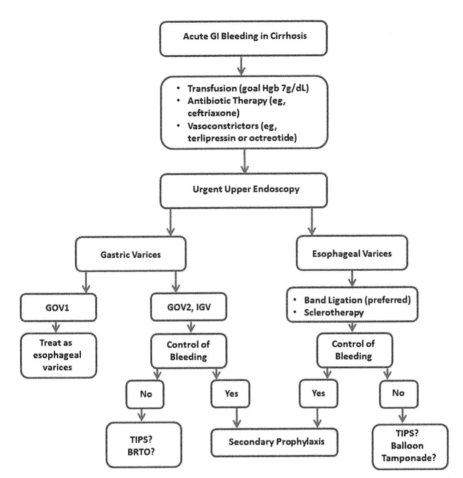

Fig. 1. A suggested algorithm for management of upper GI bleeding in patients with cirrhosis. BRTO, balloon-occluded retrograde transvenous obliteration; HgB, hemoglobin; IGV, isolated GV; TIPS, transjugular intrahepatic portosystemic shunt.

vasoactive agents is recommended and continued for 72 hours. These agents include vasopressin, somatostatin analogues (eg, octreotide), and, where available, terlipressin. These agents aid in the control of bleeding by splanchnic vasoconstriction reducing portal venous inflow and, thus, decrease portal venous pressures.

Vasopressin is a potent nonselective vasoconstrictor with widespread use in critical care. It also has been studied in treatment of variceal hemorrhage. The dose used in the treatment of variceal hemorrhage (0.2–0.4 units per minute) is considerably higher than typically used in the intensive care unit (ICU) for treatment of hypotension associated with septic shock (0.01–0.04 units per minute). Vasopressin for treatment of variceal hemorrhage has been associated with ischemic complications involving myocardium, bowel, and peripheral tissues and, therefore, should only be used for up to 24 hours.[6] Because of these side effects, several studies have examined the use of vasopressin in conjunction with nitroglycerine; in 2 randomized controlled trials comparing vasopressin alone with vasopressin plus nitroglycerine, patients who received nitroglycerine had better control of bleeding and fewer side effects.[12,13] Particularly because of its side effects, its use in this setting has fallen out of favor.

Terlipressin is a synthetic analogue of vasopressin with a longer half-life, thus, allowing it to be administered using intermittent bolus dosing, the typical dose is 2 mg intravenously (IV) every 4 hours for the first 24 hours followed by 1 mg IV every 4 hours to complete 72 hours of therapy.[14] In addition to effective control of variceal bleeding, terlipressin is the only vasoactive agent to demonstrate an improvement in survival.[15] Terlipressin is not currently available in North America.

Somatostatin or its analogues octreotide or vapreotide are alternative agents, which are also commonly used in acute variceal hemorrhage. These agents offer an improved safety profile compared with vasopressin and may safely be used for 5 days or longer in control of variceal bleeding, but their mechanism of action does not seem to be direct splanchnic vasoconstriction but rather diminished postprandial hyperemia and blunting the increase in portal pressure. Of these agents, only octreotide is available in the United States. Octreotide is typically administered as a 50-μg bolus followed by a continuous infusion of 50 μg/h. Although a meta-analysis of somatostatin analogues has not demonstrated significant benefit when used alone,[16] a separate meta-analysis of 5 studies comparing endoscopic therapy alone with endoscopic therapy plus pharmacologic agents demonstrated improved control of bleeding without differences in adverse events or mortality.[17] Although of value in the long-term management of variceal bleeding, nonselective beta-blockers have no role in the management of acute variceal bleeding.

Bacterial infection after acute upper GI bleeding occurs at a significant rate and is independently associated with the risk of early rebleeding.[18] Several studies have shown a benefit with the administration of prophylactic antibiotics in patients with cirrhosis with or without ascites and upper GI hemorrhage, establishing early antibiotic administration as the standard of care. Prophylactic administration of antibiotic therapy in patients with cirrhosis and upper GI bleeding decreases the rate of early rebleeding and increases survival.[19] Studied regimens have included oral norfloxacin (400 mg twice a day),[20] ofloxacin (200 mg twice a day either by mouth or IV),[21] and IV ceftriaxone (1 g daily). Ceftriaxone was superior to norfloxacin in prevention of infection[22]; however, local resistance patterns, drug availability (particularly an issue for norfloxacin starting in 2015), and a knowledge of recent antibiotic use should be considered when selecting an antibiotic regimen.

Once bleeding patients have been adequately resuscitated, stabilized, and appropriately intubated, urgent endoscopy with therapeutic intent should be pursued within 12 hours of admission.[23] If esophageal variceal bleeding is identified as the source of the bleeding, then preferably EVL or if necessary sclerotherapy should be carried out. Sclerotherapy is less favorable particularly because of a considerable side effect profile, including chest pain, ulceration, esophageal stricture, pleuritis, perforation, portal vein thrombosis, embolization, and bacteremia. Although other studies have shown equivalent rates of bleeding control for sclerotherapy to EVL, a randomized controlled trial in which 179 cirrhotic patients with acute esophageal variceal bleeding treated with vasoactive drugs who underwent endoscopy within 6 hours were randomized to receive sclerotherapy or EVL favored the use of EVL. Sclerotherapy was inferior to EVL in terms of initial failure to stop bleeding (15% to 4%, $P = .02$), serious side effects (13% to 4%, $P = .04$), and 6-week survival (67% to 83%, $P = .01$).

A 2002 meta-analysis demonstrated improved initial control of bleeding (relative risk [RR], 1.12; 95% CI 1.02–1.23) and 5-day hemostasis (RR 1.28; 95% CI 1.18–1.29) when combined pharmacologic and endoscopic therapy was used; there was no difference in 5-day mortality or in adverse events.[17] This finding provides a rational basis for usage of pharmacologic therapy, which can be initiated promptly in combination with EVL.

Rescue Therapies

Even with appropriate intervention, failure to control bleeding or early rebleeding occurs in up to 20% of patients with esophageal varices and 40% of patients with gastric varices. Because of the significant risk for recurrent bleeding, familiarity with and access to rescue therapies is mandatory when caring for the cirrhotic patient population. Availability of rescue therapies varies by center expertise; thus, early consideration for transfer to tertiary centers should be considered if access is locally unavailable.

Transjugular Intrahepatic Portosystemic Shunt

Placement of a transjugular intrahepatic portosystemic shunt (TIPS) is typically performed by interventional radiology specialists. In this procedure a communication is established between branches of the hepatic veins (typically the right) and the portal vein. A permanent polytetrafluoroethylene-covered stent is then left in place thereby decreasing the HVPG preferably to less than 12 mm Hg, although the magnitude of the decrease in HVPG is also of significance. TIPS has been shown to be effective as a rescue therapy in patients with difficult-to-control variceal hemorrhage. TIPS may exacerbate hepatic encephalopathy and results in increased mortality in patients who have a high model for end-stage liver disease (MELD) score[24] with the risk prohibitively high in those with MELD greater than 25. TIPS is also contraindicated in patients with other conditions, such as significant pulmonary hypertension or heart failure; thus, it must be only used in appropriately selected candidates.

Balloon Tamponade

Balloon tamponade is a rescue therapy that is effective at controlling bleeding in most patients. Typically either a Sengstaken-Blakemore or Minnesota tube is used, both of which are rubber tubes with dual esophageal and gastric balloons that apply pressure on the varices with use of traction. The former has only a gastric suction lumen, whereas the latter has both gastric and esophageal suction lumens. However, balloon tamponade is associated with a high rate of complications, including esophageal necrosis and rupture, and, therefore, is used as a temporizing measure of 24 to 48 hours in duration while awaiting definitive therapy, such as TIPS. Endotracheal intubation is mandatory in situations whereby balloon tamponade is being used.

Gastric Varices

Gastric varices (GV) occur less commonly than esophageal varices in patients with cirrhosis; though large studies are lacking, they are estimated to be present in 20% of cirrhotic patients.[25] Compared with esophageal varices, GV bleed less frequently; but when bleeding occurs, it is more severe (as reflected in transfusion requirement), is associated with a higher rate of rebleeding, and carries a higher mortality rate.[25,26]

The classification scheme for GV is based on work by Sarin and colleagues.[25] Vascular anatomy of GV is varied, and a detailed understanding of this anatomy is required to develop appropriate management techniques. GOV that extend below the gastroesophageal junction into the lesser curvature of the stomach are classified as GOV1 and are considered the same as esophageal varices with regard to vascular anatomy and management. Those that extend into the fundus of the stomach are classified GOV2. Isolated GV (IGV) are further subdivided into IGV1, which are located in the fundus, and IGV2, which are those in any other location.

Management of Bleeding Gastric Varices

General principles for initial management for bleeding GV are the same as for esophageal varices and include general resuscitative measures and initiation of pharmacologic therapy (vasoactive medications and antibiotics). Additional specific therapies are guided by location of the bleeding varix and sound knowledge of patients' vascular anatomy (see **Fig. 1**). It must be noted that large trials in management of bleeding GV are lacking at this time.

For patients who bleed from GOV2 or IGV1 type GV, endoscopic therapy with cyanoacrylate is generally accepted as the endoscopic therapy of choice,[27–29] though newer strategies have shown great promise (see later discussion). Currently, cyanoacrylate use for treatment of GV is not yet approved by the Food and Drug Administration in the United States and is limited by availability of local expertise. One large randomized prospective study of 97 patients compared gastric variceal ligation (n = 48) with cyanoacrylate injection (n = 49) for cirrhotic patients with acutely bleeding GV. The study found no difference in survival or immediate bleeding control for those with active bleeding (93% for both groups), but the 2-year and 3-year cumulative rebleeding rates were 63.1% and 72.3% for gastric variceal ligation and only 26.8% for both periods with cyanoacrylate injection (P = .01).[30] For patients with rebleeding from GV, repeat endoscopic therapy is not indicated and a move toward a more definitive therapy is recommended. In GV with refractory bleeding, TIPS may be considered early; although because of vascular anatomy, not all GV may be successfully treated with TIPS.

Balloon-occluded retrograde transvenous obliteration (BRTO) of GV is gaining popularity as a minimally invasive therapy to treat GV in the United Stated and has enjoyed widespread use in Japan since its introduction by Kanagawa and colleagues[31] in 1996 and may be superior to cyanoacrylate procedures.[32] BRTO may be considered when TIPS has relative or absolute contraindications or as a first-line treatment of GV. Successful treatment of GV with BRTO requires a detailed knowledge of the vascular anatomy of afferent and efferent vessels[27–29] and interventional radiologists skilled in the procedure. In this procedure, a balloon-tipped catheter is placed into the efferent vessel and sclerosant is injected retrograde into the varix, thus, obliterating blood flow.[33] A recent meta-analysis found that successful obliteration of GV occurs in 97% of patients treated with BRTO; major complications are rare, occurring in only 2.6% of patients.[34] Because most GV drain via a gastrorenal shunt,[33] BRTO offers the additional benefit of reduction of hepatic encephalopathy after shunt closure.[35,36] Furthermore, closure of gastrorenal shunts may increase portal venous blood flow, which improves hepatic function.[37] The increased portal venous blood flow that occurs after BRTO results in progression of esophageal varices in some cases; thus, careful screening must continue for these patients.[38,39]

DISTINCTIVE CAUSES OF NONVARICEAL GASTROINTESTINAL BLEEDING IN CIRRHOTIC PATIENTS

Nonvariceal GI bleeding may also pose significant problems for cirrhotic patients, with the two entities of portal hypertensive gastropathy (PHG) and gastric antral vascular ectasia (GAVE) being particularly notable. Although both are less likely to cause life-threatening acute bleeding than variceal causes, they may present with significant anemia, hematemesis, and melena and, thus, result in ICU admission.

The mechanisms responsible for the development of PHG are not fully understood.[40] The reported prevalence of PHG in cirrhosis varies between 20% and 80%.[41,42] Not surprising is the finding that more severe portal hypertension correlates with the presence of PHG. In a study of 254 patients with cirrhosis, independent predictors of PHG were presence of large varices, Childs-Pugh class C disease, and HVPG greater than 12 mm Hg.[43] An additional finding of this study was that patients with PHG were more likely to have deranged hemodynamic parameters as evidenced by increased cardiac output and low systemic vascular resistance.[43] Treatment of PHG depends on the patients' presentation. For patients with asymptomatic PHG, no immediate therapy is indicated. Although most often bleeding associated with PHG presents as chronic iron deficiency anemia, acute bleeding events have been reported.[44] Management of chronic PHG bleeding involves transfusion when appropriate and adequate iron replacement, and consensus guidelines recommend consideration of nonselective beta-blocker therapy.[23] In patients with acute PHG bleeding, the general approach is similar to that of variceal bleeding and includes antibiotic therapy and blood transfusion to a goal hemoglobin of 7 g/dL. In addition, 2 studies have demonstrated the efficacy of vasoactive medications octreotide[45] and terlipressin[46] in control of acute PHG-associated bleeding.

In contrast to PHG, which occurs only in the context of portal hypertension, GAVE may occur in patients without portal hypertension. The prevalence of GAVE in patients with cirrhosis is considerably lower than PHG and is estimated at 2% in patients awaiting liver transplantation.[47] Like PHG, the most common presentation is iron deficiency anemia and chronic GI blood loss. Acute bleeding is similarly uncommon. The mainstay of treatment of GAVE is argon plasma coagulation, a thermoablative technique that is applied via endoscopy. Some literature now also advocate the use of EVL in the treatment of portal hypertension–related GAVE,[48] In cases of acute hemorrhage, the approach is similar to that of other upper GI bleeding in patients with advanced liver disease (**Table 1**).

NUTRITIONAL CONCERNS AND DYSMOTILITY IN CIRRHOSIS

Protein calorie malnutrition (PCM) is common in patients with cirrhosis. PCM is found in 75% of nonhospitalized cirrhotic patients and is classified as moderate or severe in 38% of these patients.[49] The prevalence of PCM also increases with advancing states of disease; in this same study, 21% of patients with Childs-Pugh class A disease had moderate to severe PCM compared with 58% of patients with Childs-Pugh class C.[49] When present, PCM contributes to increased prevalence of complications, such as ascites and hepatorenal syndrome, increased length of stay, and a 2-fold increase in hospital mortality.[50]

There are many features of cirrhosis that contribute to the development of PCM (**Fig. 2**). To begin with, nutrient intake is impaired in cirrhosis through a variety of mechanisms. The development of ascites decreases postprandial gastric volumes, impairs gastric accommodation, and diminishes caloric intake as compared with healthy controls; all of these effects are reversed by performance of large volume paracentesis.[51] Prolonged small bowel transit times and impaired small bowel motility may contribute to small bowel bacterial overgrowth all of which have been associated with portal hypertension contributing to impaired nutrient absorption.[52] Although not uniformly present in portal hypertension, increased intestinal hyperpermeability has been shown in the setting of portal hypertension and ascites[53] and may be associated with nutrient loss and bacterial translocation. It is also likely that hepatic encephalopathy also contributes to poor oral intake. Finally, iatrogenic contributions to malnutrition in hospitalized patients are common; misconceptions regarding the use of protein restrictions in encephalopathic patients and maintaining nothing-by-mouth status for procedures further exacerbate caloric deficiencies in hospitalized cirrhotic patients.[54]

Table 1
Management of gastrointestinal bleeding in patients with cirrhosis

Bleeding Source	Initial Actions	Definitive Measures	Rescue Therapies
Esophageal varices	• Vasoconstrictors ○ Terlipressin 2 mg IV q 4 h × 24 h followed by 1 mg IV q 4 h to complete 72 h of therapy OR ○ Octreotide 50-μg bolus followed by infusion of 50 μg/ h × 72 h PLUS • Antibiotics ○ IV ceftriaxone 1 g daily × 7 d OR ○ Oral or IV quinolone × 7 d	• Endoscopic variceal band ligation • TIPS • Liver transplantation	• Balloon tamponade • TIPS
GV	Same as above for esophageal varices	• Endoscopic band ligation • Cyanoacrylate injection • BRTO • Liver transplantation	• Balloon tamponade • TIPS • BRTO
PHG, acute	Same as above for esophageal varices	TIPS? Liver transplantation	TIPS?
GAVE, acute	Same as above for esophageal varices	Argon plasma coagulation	N/A
PHG, chronic	Transfusion as appropriate Iron replacement (may require IV)	Liver transplantation	N/A
GAVE, chronic	Same as for chronic PHG	Argon plasma coagulation	N/A

With advancing liver dysfunction, metabolic abnormalities further contribute to exacerbation in nutritional deficiencies due to increased energy expenditure and catabolism of protein stores. Between 15% and 30% of patients with cirrhosis have been shown to be hypermetabolic as defined by a resting energy expenditure of greater than 120% of predicted; the mechanisms responsible for this phenomenon are not well understood.[55,56] With advancing fibrosis, the functional hepatocyte mass decreases resulting in impaired hepatic glycogen metabolism, thus, promoting gluconeogenesis from alternative fuel sources, such as protein and fat. Patients with cirrhosis are susceptible to the effects of even brief fasting; as one study demonstrated after a brief overnight fast, patients with cirrhosis had rates of protein and fat catabolism equal to healthy controls who had fasted for 2 to 3 days.[57]

Macronutrient deficiencies are commonly due to poor dietary intake, fat malabsorption in cholestatic liver disease, and diuretic use.[58] Deficiencies in vitamins A and D are the most commonly reported.[58] Thiamine deficiency is frequently underappreciated in patients with cirrhosis and may have important implications in this population. In an

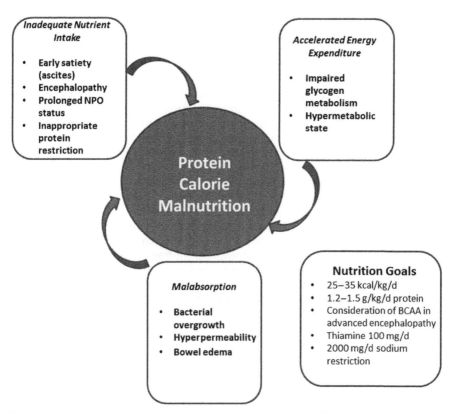

Fig. 2. Contributors to malnutrition in cirrhosis and basic nutritional recommendations. BCAA, branched chain amino acid; NPO, nothing by mouth.

autopsy study by Kril and Butterworth,[59] 50% of patients with cirrhosis due to alcohol and 50% of patients with cirrhosis from non–alcohol-related diseases had pathologic evidence of thiamine deficiency. Butterworth[60] has further described a mechanism by which elevated levels of ammonia coupled with thiamine deficiency may act through a synergistic mechanism to exacerbate diencephalic and cerebellar symptoms contributing to neurologic dysfunction. Because thiamine replacement is inexpensive and safe, and because prolonged thiamine deficiency may result in irreversible brain lesions, the authors recommend early thiamine replacement in critically ill patients with cirrhosis. Absorption of thiamine by the oral route is inefficient[61] and may be further impaired in critically ill patients and particularly in patients with alcohol-related cirrhosis.[62,63] Parenteral administration is recommended in critically ill cirrhotic patients; although optimal dosing has not been established, the authors recommend dosages of 100 mg/d for 3 to 5 days.

General recommendations for nutritional support of cirrhotic patients are designed with the goal of addressing the nutritional complications described earlier. The European Society for Clinical Nutrition and Metabolism (ESPEN) and the American Society of Parenteral and Enteral Nutrition (ASPEN) have both published recommendations for nutritional supplementation in cirrhosis. The ESPEN's recommendations are for a goal of 35 to 40 kcal/kg/d with 1.2 to 1.5 g/kg/d protein.[64] The ASPEN's guidelines recommend a goal of 25 to 35 kcal/kg/d in patients without hepatic encephalopathy and

35 kcal/kg/d for patients with encephalopathy.[65] Protein restriction should not be used even in the setting of hepatic encephalopathy. Furthermore, it is recommended that enteral nutritional supplementation be initiated when malnutrition and/or inadequate caloric intake is recognized[64]; for critically ill cirrhotic patients this is typically on presentation to the ICU. Early tube feeding is recommended in patients who are not able to meet caloric goals via the oral route; it is important to note that the presence of esophageal varices is not a contraindication to enteric tube placement. Placement of percutaneous feeding tubes is generally contraindicated in patients with cirrhosis because of associated complications and should be avoided.[64] For patients who have contraindications to enteral feeding that have persisted for greater than 72 hours, parenteral nutritional supplementation should be considered.[66]

Whole protein supplements are generally preferred; however, the use of branched chain amino acid (BCAA) formulas has been the subject of study. Current guidelines from the ESPEN recommend consideration of BCAA-enriched formulas in patients with problematic encephalopathy based on 2 randomized controlled trials that have demonstrated that long-term administration (12–24 months) results in delayed progression of hepatic failure and improvement in event-free survival.[67,68] The biochemical basis for the recommendation of BCAA supplementation is related to the impact on pathogenesis of hepatic encephalopathy. BCAA supplementation may improve hepatic encephalopathy by stimulating synthesis of glutamine from ammonia and glutamate in skeletal muscle and by decreasing tryptophan accumulation in the brain.[65] Because BCAA supplements are expensive and poorly tolerated, they have yet to gain widespread usage.

SUMMARY

Cirrhosis results in numerous systemic complications. GI complications are frequent and result in significant morbidity and mortality. For patients who present to the ICU, a multidisciplinary approach is typically required for the management of these complicated patients. The approach to management often times will be guided by local expertise. In centers with limited access to advanced endoscopy and interventional radiology techniques, early referral to a tertiary care center, preferably one with transplant expertise, is warranted. Ensuring that patients have appropriate follow-up with hepatology further ensures that long-term management of GI complications are properly addressed. With appropriate screening and preventive treatment, many GI complications may be avoided and their impact minimized.

REFERENCES

1. Bhathal PS, Grossman HJ. Reduction of the increased portal vascular resistance of the isolated perfused cirrhotic rat liver by vasodilators. J Hepatol 1985;1(4):325–37.
2. Gupta TK, Toruner M, Chung MK, et al. Endothelial dysfunction and decreased production of nitric oxide in the intrahepatic microcirculation of cirrhotic rats. Hepatology 1998;28(4):926–31.
3. Mittal MK, Gupta TK, Lee FY, et al. Nitric oxide modulates hepatic vascular tone in normal rat liver. Am J Physiol 1994;267(3 Pt 1):G416–22.
4. Frances R, Munoz C, Zapater P, et al. Bacterial DNA activates cell mediated immune response and nitric oxide overproduction in peritoneal macrophages from patients with cirrhosis and ascites. Gut 2004;53(6):860–4.
5. Wiest R, Groszmann RJ. Nitric oxide and portal hypertension: its role in the regulation of intrahepatic and splanchnic vascular resistance. Semin Liver Dis 1999; 19(4):411–26.

6. Garcia-Tsao G, Sanyal AJ, Grace ND, et al, Practice Guidelines Committee of the American Association for the Study of Liver Diseases, Practice Parameters Committee of the American College of Gastroenterology. Prevention and management of gastroesophageal varices and variceal hemorrhage in cirrhosis. Hepatology 2007;46(3):922–38.

7. Merli M, Nicolini G, Angeloni S, et al. Incidence and natural history of small esophageal varices in cirrhotic patients. J Hepatol 2003;38(3):266–72.

8. Groszmann RJ, Garcia-Tsao G, Bosch J, et al. Beta-blockers to prevent gastroesophageal varices in patients with cirrhosis. N Engl J Med 2005;353(21): 2254–61.

9. Groszmann RJ, Wongcharatrawee S. The hepatic venous pressure gradient: anything worth doing should be done right. Hepatology 2004;39(2):280–2.

10. Chalasani N, Kahi C, Francois F, et al. Improved patient survival after acute variceal bleeding: a multicenter, cohort study. Am J Gastroenterol 2003;98(3):653–9.

11. Villanueva C, Colomo A, Bosch A, et al. Transfusion strategies for acute upper gastrointestinal bleeding. N Engl J Med 2013;368(1):11–21.

12. Gimson AE, Westaby D, Hegarty J, et al. A randomized trial of vasopressin and vasopressin plus nitroglycerin in the control of acute variceal hemorrhage. Hepatology 1986;6(3):410–3.

13. Tsai YT, Lay CS, Lai KH, et al. Controlled trial of vasopressin plus nitroglycerin vs. vasopressin alone in the treatment of bleeding esophageal varices. Hepatology 1986;6(3):406–9.

14. Burroughs AK. Pharmacological treatment of acute variceal bleeding. Digestion 1998;59(Suppl 2):28–36.

15. Ioannou GN, Doust J, Rockey DC. Systematic review: terlipressin in acute oesophageal variceal haemorrhage. Aliment Pharmacol Ther 2003;17(1):53–64.

16. Gotzsche PC, Hrobjartsson A. Somatostatin analogues for acute bleeding oesophageal varices. Cochrane Database Syst Rev 2008;(3):CD000193.

17. Banares R, Albillos A, Rincon D, et al. Endoscopic treatment versus endoscopic plus pharmacologic treatment for acute variceal bleeding: a meta-analysis. Hepatology 2002;35(3):609–15.

18. Goulis J, Armonis A, Patch D, et al. Bacterial infection is independently associated with failure to control bleeding in cirrhotic patients with gastrointestinal hemorrhage. Hepatology 1998;27(5):1207–12.

19. Bernard B, Grange JD, Khac EN, et al. Antibiotic prophylaxis for the prevention of bacterial infections in cirrhotic patients with gastrointestinal bleeding: a meta-analysis. Hepatology 1999;29(6):1655–61.

20. Rimola A, Garcia-Tsao G, Navasa M, et al. Diagnosis, treatment and prophylaxis of spontaneous bacterial peritonitis: a consensus document. International Ascites Club. J Hepatol 2000;32(1):142–53.

21. Hou MC, Lin HC, Liu TT, et al. Antibiotic prophylaxis after endoscopic therapy prevents rebleeding in acute variceal hemorrhage: a randomized trial. Hepatology 2004;39(3):746–53.

22. Fernandez J, Ruiz del Arbol L, Gomez C, et al. Norfloxacin vs ceftriaxone in the prophylaxis of infections in patients with advanced cirrhosis and hemorrhage. Gastroenterology 2006;131(4):1049–56 [quiz: 1285].

23. de Franchis R, Baveno VIF. Expanding consensus in portal hypertension: report of the Baveno VI Consensus Workshop: stratifying risk and individualizing care for portal hypertension. J Hepatol 2015;63(3):743–52.

24. Malinchoc M, Kamath PS, Gordon FD, et al. A model to predict poor survival in patients undergoing transjugular intrahepatic portosystemic shunts. Hepatology 2000;31(4):864–71.

25. Sarin SK, Lahoti D, Saxena SP, et al. Prevalence, classification and natural history of gastric varices: a long-term follow-up study in 568 portal hypertension patients. Hepatology 1992;16(6):1343–9.

26. de Franchis R, Primignani M. Natural history of portal hypertension in patients with cirrhosis. Clin Liver Dis 2001;5(3):645–63.

27. Lo GH, Lai KH, Cheng JS, et al. A prospective, randomized trial of butyl cyano-acrylate injection versus band ligation in the management of bleeding gastric varices. Hepatology 2001;33(5):1060–4.

28. Oho K, Iwao T, Sumino M, et al. Ethanolamine oleate versus butyl cyanoacrylate for bleeding gastric varices: a nonrandomized study. Endoscopy 1995;27(5): 349–54.

29. Sarin SK, Jain AK, Jain M, et al. A randomized controlled trial of cyanoacrylate versus alcohol injection in patients with isolated fundic varices. Am J Gastroen-terol 2002;97(4):1010–5.

30. Tan PC, Hou MC, Lin HC, et al. A randomized trial of endoscopic treatment of acute gastric variceal hemorrhage: N-butyl-2-cyanoacrylate injection versus band ligation. Hepatology 2006;43(4):690–7.

31. Kanagawa H, Mima S, Kouyama H, et al. Treatment of gastric fundal varices by balloon-occluded retrograde transvenous obliteration. J Gastroenterol Hepatol 1996;11(1):51–8.

32. Hong CH, Kim HJ, Park JH, et al. Treatment of patients with gastric variceal hem-orrhage: endoscopic N-butyl-2-cyanoacrylate injection versus balloon-occluded retrograde transvenous obliteration. J Gastroenterol Hepatol 2009;24(3):372–8.

33. Kiyosue H, Mori H, Matsumoto S, et al. Transcatheter obliteration of gastric vari-ces. Part 1. Anatomic classification. Radiographics 2003;23(4):911–20.

34. Park JK, Saab S, Kee ST, et al. Balloon-occluded retrograde transvenous obliter-ation (BRTO) for treatment of gastric varices: review and meta-analysis. Dig Dis Sci 2015;60(6):1543–53.

35. Gwon DI, Ko GY, Yoon HK, et al. Gastric varices and hepatic encephalopathy: treatment with vascular plug and gelatin sponge-assisted retrograde transvenous obliteration–a primary report. Radiology 2013;268(1):281–7.

36. Fukuda T, Hirota S, Sugimura K. Long-term results of balloon-occluded retro-grade transvenous obliteration for the treatment of gastric varices and hepatic encephalopathy. J Vasc Interv Radiol 2001;12(3):327–36.

37. Miyamoto Y, Oho K, Kumamoto M, et al. Balloon-occluded retrograde transve-nous obliteration improves liver function in patients with cirrhosis and portal hy-pertension. J Gastroenterol Hepatol 2003;18(8):934–42.

38. Chikamori F, Kuniyoshi N, Shibuya S, et al. Combination treatment of transjugular retrograde obliteration and endoscopic embolization for portosystemic encepha-lopathy with esophageal varices. Hepato Gastroenterology 2004;51(59):1379–81.

39. Ninoi T, Nishida N, Kaminou T, et al. Balloon-occluded retrograde transvenous obliteration of gastric varices with gastrorenal shunt: long-term follow-up in 78 pa-tients. AJR Am J Roentgenol 2005;184(4):1340–6.

40. Ferraz JG, Wallace JL. Underlying mechanisms of portal hypertensive gastropa-thy. J Clin Gastroenterol 1997;25(Suppl 1):S73–8.

41. Primignani M, Carpinelli L, Preatoni P, et al. Natural history of portal hypertensive gastropathy in patients with liver cirrhosis. The New Italian Endoscopic Club for

the study and treatment of esophageal varices (NIEC). Gastroenterology 2000; 119(1):181–7.

42. Ripoll C, Garcia-Tsao G. The management of portal hypertensive gastropathy and gastric antral vascular ectasia. Dig Liver Dis 2011;43(5):345–51.

43. Kumar A, Mishra SR, Sharma P, et al. Clinical, laboratory, and hemodynamic parameters in portal hypertensive gastropathy: a study of 254 cirrhotics. J Clin Gastroenterol 2010;44(4):294–300.

44. Gostout CJ, Viggiano TR, Balm RK. Acute gastrointestinal bleeding from portal hypertensive gastropathy: prevalence and clinical features. Am J Gastroenterol 1993;88(12):2030–3.

45. Zhou Y, Qiao L, Wu J, et al. Comparison of the efficacy of octreotide, vasopressin, and omeprazole in the control of acute bleeding in patients with portal hypertensive gastropathy: a controlled study. J Gastroenterol Hepatol 2002;17(9):973–9.

46. Bruha R, Marecek Z, Spicak J, et al. Double-blind randomized, comparative multicenter study of the effect of terlipressin in the treatment of acute esophageal variceal and/or hypertensive gastropathy bleeding. Hepatogastroenterology 2002;49(46):1161–6.

47. Ward EM, Raimondo M, Rosser BG, et al. Prevalence and natural history of gastric antral vascular ectasia in patients undergoing orthotopic liver transplantation. J Clin Gastroenterol 2004;38(10):898–900.

48. Keohane J, Berro W, Harewood GC, et al. Band ligation of gastric antral vascular ectasia is a safe and effective endoscopic treatment. Dig Endosc 2013;25(4): 392–6.

49. Carvalho L, Parise ER. Evaluation of nutritional status of nonhospitalized patients with liver cirrhosis. Arq Gastroenterol 2006;43(4):269–74.

50. Sam J, Nguyen GC. Protein-calorie malnutrition as a prognostic indicator of mortality among patients hospitalized with cirrhosis and portal hypertension. Liver Int 2009;29(9):1396–402.

51. Aqel BA, Scolapio JS, Dickson RC, et al. Contribution of ascites to impaired gastric function and nutritional intake in patients with cirrhosis and ascites. Clin Gastroenterol Hepatol 2005;3(11):1095–100.

52. Gunnarsdottir SA, Sadik R, Shev S, et al. Small intestinal motility disturbances and bacterial overgrowth in patients with liver cirrhosis and portal hypertension. Am J Gastroenterol 2003;98(6):1362–70.

53. Zuckerman MJ, Menzies IS, Ho H, et al. Assessment of intestinal permeability and absorption in cirrhotic patients with ascites using combined sugar probes. Dig Dis Sci 2004;49(4):621–6.

54. Plauth M, Schutz ET. Cachexia in liver cirrhosis. Int J Cardiol 2002;85(1):83–7.

55. Muller MJ, Bottcher J, Selberg O, et al. Hypermetabolism in clinically stable patients with liver cirrhosis. Am J Clin Nutr 1999;69(6):1194–201.

56. Peng S, Plank LD, McCall JL, et al. Body composition, muscle function, and energy expenditure in patients with liver cirrhosis: a comprehensive study. Am J Clin Nutr 2007;85(5):1257–66.

57. Owen OE, Reichle FA, Mozzoli MA, et al. Hepatic, gut, and renal substrate flux rates in patients with hepatic cirrhosis. J Clin Invest 1981;68(1):240–52.

58. Cheung K, Lee SS, Raman M. Prevalence and mechanisms of malnutrition in patients with advanced liver disease, and nutrition management strategies. Clin Gastroenterol Hepatol 2012;10(2):117–25.

59. Kril JJ, Butterworth RF. Diencephalic and cerebellar pathology in alcoholic and nonalcoholic patients with end-stage liver disease. Hepatology 1997;26(4): 837–41.

60. Butterworth RF. Thiamine deficiency-related brain dysfunction in chronic liver failure. Metab Brain Dis 2009;24(1):189–96.
61. Friedemann TE, Kmieciak TC, Keegan P, et al. The absorption, destruction, and excretion of orally administered thiamin by human subjects. Gastroenterology 1948;11(1):100–14.
62. Hoyumpa AM Jr, Nichols S, Henderson GI, et al. Intestinal thiamin transport: effect of chronic ethanol administration in rats. Am J Clin Nutr 1978;31(6):938–45.
63. Thomson AD, Baker H, Leevy CM. Patterns of 35S-thiamine hydrochloride absorption in the malnourished alcoholic patient. J Lab Clin Med 1970;76(1):34–45.
64. Plauth M, Cabre E, Riggio O, et al. Espen guidelines on enteral nutrition: liver disease. Clin Nutr 2006;25(2):285–94.
65. Juakiem W, Torres DM, Harrison SA. Nutrition in cirrhosis and chronic liver disease. Clin Liver Dis 2014;18(1):179–90.
66. Plauth M, Cabre E, Campillo B, et al, ESPEN. ESPEN guidelines on parenteral nutrition: hepatology. Clin Nutr 2009;28(4):436–44.
67. Marchesini G, Bianchi G, Merli M, et al. Nutritional supplementation with branched-chain amino acids in advanced cirrhosis: a double-blind, randomized trial. Gastroenterology 2003;124(7):1792–801.
68. Muto Y, Sato S, Watanabe A, et al. Effects of oral branched-chain amino acid granules on event-free survival in patients with liver cirrhosis. Clin Gastroenterol Hepatol 2005;3(7):705–13.

Hematological Issues in Liver Disease

Michael G. Allison, MD[a],*, Carl B. Shanholtz, MD[b], Ashutosh Sachdeva, MBBS[c]

KEYWORDS

- Cirrhosis • Acute liver failure • Thrombocytopenia • Coagulopathy • Thrombosis
- Anticoagulation

KEY POINTS

- The international normalized ratio (INR) should not be used as a measure of coagulation status in patients with liver failure.
- Liver failure results in a state of "rebalanced hemostasis" marked by a decrease in both procoagulation and anticoagulation factors.
- Patients with liver disease are not auto anticoagulated.
- Hospitalized patients with liver disease have high thrombotic risk and should receive pharmacologic antithrombotic prophylaxis in the absence of contraindications.
- Patients with liver disease undergoing invasive procedures should have appropriate platelet counts for the proposed procedure. The best approach to manage elevations in INR is unclear.

INTRODUCTION

Hepatic dysfunction results in complex hematologic abnormalities; the pathophysiological basis of these abnormalities are frequently misunderstood and may lead to suboptimal management. Diagnostic criteria for liver failure include elevation in the international normalized ratio (INR). Using elevations in conventional assays for anticoagulation monitoring has resulted in the assumption that liver disease, both acute and chronic, is a state of hypocoagulability, marked by a predilection for bleeding diatheses. Recent investigations into the coagulation milieu have elucidated that many patients with underlying acute or chronic liver dysfunction do not have evidence of auto-anticoagulation.[1] Counterintuitively, patients actually have disorders of the coagulation system that result in normal coagulation, or sometimes even a hypercoagulable

Disclosures: The authors have no financial disclosures to report.
[a] Critical Care Medicine, St. Agnes Hospital, 900 South Caton Avenue, Box 062, Baltimore, MD 21229, USA; [b] Medical Intensive Care Unit, Division of Pulmonary and Critical Care, University of Maryland School of Medicine, 110 South Paca Street, 2nd Floor, Baltimore, MD 21201, USA; [c] Interventional Pulmonary Program, Division of Pulmonary and Critical Care, University of Maryland School of Medicine, 110 South Paca Street, 2nd Floor, Baltimore, MD 21201, USA
* Corresponding author.
E-mail address: mgallison@gmail.com

Crit Care Clin 32 (2016) 385–396
http://dx.doi.org/10.1016/j.ccc.2016.03.004
0749-0704/16/$ – see front matter © 2016 Elsevier Inc. All rights reserved.

state that can clinically manifest with thrombotic complications. Bleeding diathesis that occur in patients hospitalized with acute liver failure (ALF) and cirrhosis are more likely attributable to the hemodynamic consequences of liver disease, such as increased portal and splanchnic pressures. In recent years, it has become evident that appropriately assessing patients for the risk of bleeding and thrombosis cannot be done with traditional measures of coagulation, such as prothrombin time (PT), partial thromboplastin time (PTT), or INR. In this context, there is now an emerging role for viscoelastic testing to determine the risk of bleeding and guide blood product replacement therapy in patients with liver disease. Further, prophylaxis against thrombosis, treatment of thrombosis, and transfusion of blood products to treat bleeding requires knowledge of the alterations of the hematologic system specific to patients with liver disease. In this article, we discuss mechanisms for the coagulation abnormalities, comment on the limitations of laboratory testing, and review clinical manifestations of hematological alterations in patients with acute and/or chronic liver disease.

MECHANISMS OF HEMATOLOGIC ABNORMALITIES IN LIVER FAILURE

There has been considerable refinement in the understanding of the coagulation changes occurring in liver failure in the past 10 years. A disease traditionally thought to result in an anticoagulated state that places patients at increased risk of bleeding has now been recategorized. "Rebalanced hemostasis" is the term that has been used to describe the coagulation abnormalities specific to liver disease, wherein there is a commensurate fall in coagulation proteins that counterbalance the decrease in the factors that promote coagulation.[1] This balance is tenuous, as patients with liver disease can present with complications of both bleeding and thrombosis. Although there are differences between the hematologic abnormalities in ALF and chronic liver disease with cirrhosis, both manifest adaptations for achieving a rebalanced state (**Table 1**). A new balance is reached with procoagulation factors, anticoagulant factors, platelets, von Willebrand factor (vWF), and fibrinolysis.

Coagulation Factors

The liver is responsible for synthesizing most of the proteins that control the coagulation system. This includes procoagulant factors (F) I (fibrinogen), II (prothrombin), V, VII, IX, X, XI, XII, XIIIa, and also includes the anticoagulants protein C, protein S, and antithrombin. In hepatic dysfunction, levels of these factors are decreased, but

Table 1 Rebalanced hemostasis in acute liver failure compared with cirrhosis		
	Acute Liver Failure	Cirrhosis
Anticoagulants		
Protein C/S	↓	↓
Antithrombin	↓	↓
Procoagulants		
Coagulation factors	↓↓	↓
Factor VIII	↑	↑
Fibrinogen	↓	↓↓
Platelets	↓	↓
Von Willebrand Factor	↑	↑

Abbreviations: ↑, protein factors are up-regulated in disease; ↓, protein factors are down-regulated in disease; Protein C/S, protein C/protein S.

the decrease in anticoagulant proteins approximates the decrease in procoagulants such that a state of balance is achieved.[2,3] FVIII and vWF are the notable procoagulants that are elevated in liver disease.[4] The elevation of FVIII level occurs in states of acute and chronic liver failure due to the combined effects of increased production by the endothelial system and decreased plasma clearance secondary to increased concentrations of vWF that stabilize FVIII.[5] These elevations of FVIII and vWF play a crucial role in rebalancing the hemostatic system when coagulation factors produced by hepatocytes are decreased.

Platelets

Platelets are an important part of primary hemostasis, and they are often quantitatively decreased in liver failure. Development of thrombocytopenia in patients with acute and/or chronic liver disease is multifactorial. With rising portal pressures during liver failure, the spleen becomes a repository for sequestration. In advanced stages of liver failure and hepatocyte loss, production of thrombopoietin by hepatocytes is diminished, causing suppression of platelet production in the bone marrow. Parenteral thrombopoietin is effective in raising the platelet count in clinical trials but has an associated increased thrombotic risk.[6,7] In the laboratory setting, low platelet counts have been found to produce less thrombin for clot formation than samples with higher platelet counts.[3] In addition to quantitatively low platelet counts, a functional platelet defect exists and the resultant prolongation in bleeding time is closely related to degree of liver failure.[8,9] Nevertheless, adaptations occur to overcome the quantitative deficiency in platelet count, as discussed in the subsequent section.

Von Willebrand Factor

During normal coagulation, vWF plays a major role in promoting primary hemostasis by facilitating platelet adherence. Additionally, vWF circulates in the blood bound to FVIII, which is upregulated in liver failure as previously mentioned, allowing this factor to remain in its active state. In states of liver failure, vWF is also upregulated due to increased production by endothelial cells.[10,11] High levels of vWF act to preserve a normal state of platelet function in the setting of a low total platelet count.

Fibrinolysis

In a normally functioning coagulation system, fibrinogen is enzymatically converted by thrombin into fibrin. Fibrin is cross-linked on platelets and stabilized by FXIII. Clot formation is a dynamic process in which there is coexisting dissolution of the fibrin strands through fibrinolysis. In liver disease, the concept of primary hyperfibrinolysis and premature clot dissolution has been described for more than a century.[12] Laboratory analysis has supported this assertion by finding derangements in the individual components of the fibrinolytic system. Fibrinogen is produced by hepatocytes, and decreased levels of fibrinogen may reflect decreased production. Tissue plasminogen activator (tPA), the main promoter of fibrinolysis, is upregulated in acute and chronic liver failure. Plasminogen, antiplasmin, and thrombin activatable fibrinolysis inhibitor, which compose the antifibrinolytic pathway, are reduced. These changes would suggest that the fibrinolytic system is tipped toward hyperfibrinolysis, but assays that directly measure clot lysis fail to demonstrate a fibrinolytic state in patients with cirrhosis.[13,14] Studies in patients with ALF have surprisingly shown a state of hypofibrinolysis.[15] This has led experts to speculate that there may be a rebalancing of the fibrinolytic system in liver disease, with a resultant balance that may easily be perturbed toward acquired fibrinolysis.[16]

DIAGNOSING HEMATOLOGIC ABNORMALITIES

Diagnosing the hematologic abnormalities and quantifying of the state of rebalanced hemostasis discussed previously is difficult to capture with traditional assessments of coagulation. PT, PTT, and INR provide information about how intrinsic procoagulants may be diminished toward a state of anticoagulation, but do not provide information on how intrinsic anticoagulants (protein C, protein S, and antithrombin) may be similarly diminished toward a state of balanced procoagulation. Traditional coagulation assays are inadequate to assess bleeding risk in patients with liver disease and may result in the inappropriate use of blood products in patients who have little to no bleeding risk.

In the research laboratory setting, tests that assess the simultaneous presence of anticoagulants and procoagulants have been used to better understand the hemostatic changes in liver disease. One such test is the thrombin generation assay, which uses recombinant tissue factor to measure the effective thrombin generation when both anticoagulants and procoagulants are activated. When plasma of a patient with cirrhosis is compared with normal controls in this manner, the endogenous thrombin potential (ETP) is the same.[2,3] Although there is promise in ETP testing, one study found poor ability of this test to discriminate between patients who had bleeding or thrombotic events.[15] The bedside clinical utility of such tests has not yet been validated.

Viscoelastic testing has shown promise in quantifying the entire clot-forming process in patients with liver failure. Unlike ETP, viscoelastic testing, known commercially as thromboelastography (TEG) or rotational thromboelastometry (ROTEM), is becoming more widely available to clinicians in academic centers or large community referral centers. Whole blood is sampled and a recording of the dynamics of clot formation, strength, and stability provides an overall assessment of hemostasis (**Table 2**). The first use of TEG in patients with liver disease was to guide blood product resuscitation in patients undergoing orthotopic liver transplantation. When used, TEG parameters resulted in fewer transfusions of blood and fresh frozen plasma (FFP) with increased use of platelets and cryoprecipitate.[17] In patients with ALF who were not yet actively listed for transplantation, TEG demonstrated a normal coagulation profile in 63% and a hypercoagulable profile in 8% of patients.[18] TEG has been assessed in patients with cirrhosis as well, demonstrating that patients with stable cirrhosis have maximal amplitude (MA) values within normal limits, but that the MA was lower in patients with more advanced disease.[19] The lower maximal amplitude may represent a tendency toward anticoagulation, as MA is a measure of maximal clot firmness as depicted in **Fig. 1** and **Table 2**. A representative case is presented in **Fig. 2**, discussing the potential role of TEG in the clinical setting. ROTEM also has been studied in patients with stable cirrhosis, and there were correlations in the abnormalities seen on ROTEM with some abnormalities seen on traditional markers of coagulation.[20] Viscoelastic testing holds promise for improved quantification of the coagulation status of patients with liver disease and remains an active area of investigation.

Given the ability of TEG to demonstrate normal hemostatic parameters in patients with both acute and chronic liver disease, investigators have become interested in determining whether TEG has the ability to predict if patients are more likely to have clinical bleeding or thrombotic events. In patients with ALF, the TEG R-time was prolonged in patients with clinical bleeding, whereas the INR was not significantly different in the bleeding and nonbleeding groups.[18] A study in patients with cirrhosis found that TEG could predict which patients would re-bleed from esophageal varices, whereas traditional coagulation parameters failed to predict bleeding events.[21]

Table 2
Interpretation of thromboelastogram (TEG)

TEG Measurement	Abbreviation	Definition	Interpretation and Suggested Replacement Product
Reaction time, min	R or r	Time from initiation of coagulation to fibrin formation	Prolonged R represents deficiency of clotting factors. Suggest fresh frozen plasma.
Kinetic time, min	K or k	Time from formation of fibrin to 20 mm of clot strength	Prolonged K represents deficiency of fibrinogen. Suggest cryoprecipitate.
Alpha-angle, degrees	Angle	Rate of fibrin formation	Decreased angle represents deficiency of fibrinogen. Suggest cryoprecipitate.
Maximum amplitude, mm	MA	Maximum clot strength	Decreased MA represents low platelet function. Suggest platelet transfusion.
Lysis-30, %	Ly-30	Fibrinolysis 30 minutes after MA	Increased Ly-30 may be amenable to aminocaproic acid or tranexamic acid to prevent clot lysis.

Data from Stravitz RT. Potential applications of thromboelastography in patients with acute and chronic liver disease. Gastroenterol Hepatol (N Y) 2012;8:515.

Despite the knowledge gained about the hemostatic status of patients with liver disease, viscoelastic testing in these patients should be ordered and interpreted with caution. Many of these studies examined the correlation between clinical bleeding and laboratory parameters in a retrospective manner. Some studies even have

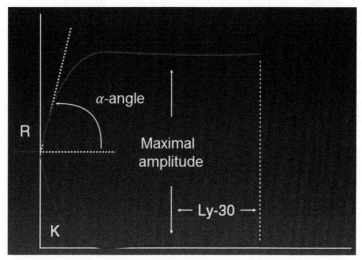

Fig. 1. Schematic representation of thromboelastogram. A normal thromboelastogram displaying individual parameters. See **Table 2** for interpretation. K, kinetic time; Ly-30, clot lysis in 30 minutes; R, reaction time.

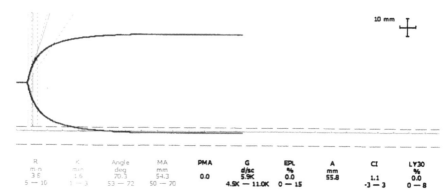

R	K	Angle	MA	PMA	G	EPL	A	CI	LY30
min	min	deg	mm		d/sc	%	mm		%
3.5	1.6	70.3	54.3	0.0	5.9K	0.0	55.8	1.1	0.0
5 — 10	1 — 3	53 — 72	50 — 70		4.5K — 11.0K	0 — 15		-3 — 3	0 — 8

Fig. 2. Clinical case representing utility of thromboelastography in liver disease. TEG performed in a 39-year-old patient with massive hematemesis from variceal bleeding. TEG was performed to guide resuscitation after 4 bands were endoscopically placed. The INR was 1.7, the platelet count was 66 K/µL, and the fibrinogen level was 178 mg/dL. No further blood products were given. As evidenced by the short R-time, the patient was likely hypercoagulable after his initial resuscitation. A, amplitude; CI, coagulation index; EPL, estimated percent lysis; G, G parameter; PMA, platelet mapping assay.

contradictory findings that are not easily explained. In early studies by Kang and colleagues,[17] the TEG parameters correlated well with conventional assays of coagulation such as INR. More recently, Stravitz and colleagues[18] found correlation between clinically evident thrombosis and a prolonged R-time on TEG, a value that reflects hypocoagulability and not hypercoagulability. Well-designed, randomized, prospective studies to clarify the ability of TEG to assess the bleeding risk or thrombotic risk as compared with conventional tests of hemostasis are needed.

CLINICAL IMPLICATIONS OF COAGULOPATHY OF LIVER DISEASE
Bleeding

A high percentage of patients with cirrhosis present to acute care with a bleeding diathesis. Variceal bleeding is the most common and concerning type of bleed, occurring in 25% to 35% of patients with cirrhosis.[22] Nonvariceal bleeding is almost equally common, noted in 20% of patients admitted with decompensated cirrhosis.[23] To date, no test has convincingly been able to predict the risk of bleeding in patients with liver disease. The bleeding time, platelet counts, and fibrinogen level all have little predictive value. The INR has failed to predict bleeding risk in patients receiving liver biopsy, paracentesis, bronchoscopy, central venous catheter placement, and coronary artery catheterization.[24–29] Because patients do not demonstrate a correlation between traditional coagulation parameters and bleeding, investigators have hypothesized that forces other than those involved in hemostasis instead drive the bleeding risk. The presence of portal hypertension, infection, or renal dysfunction has association with bleeding events in patients with cirrhosis. Patients with ALF are unlikely to bleed and often do not have evidence of portal hypertensive changes.

Disseminated Intravascular Coagulation and Accelerated Intravascular Coagulation and Fibrinolysis

Alterations in fibrinogen levels and/or function are features of advanced liver disease. The clinical implications of these alterations are widely discussed and debated. Patients with liver failure can exhibit a clinical syndrome similar to disseminated intravascular coagulation (DIC) called accelerated intravascular coagulation and fibrinolysis (AICF).[30] The fibrinogen count is typically less than 120 mg/dL in patients with AICF and it is clinically seen as oozing from puncture sites or indwelling catheter sites. Adding further confusion to states of low fibrinogen, patients with liver disease can develop overt DIC or an overlap of AICF and DIC.[30] Although FVIII levels are elevated in AICF and decreased in DIC, the differentiation between these 2 syndromes is difficult to determine and there is not a gold standard test available to date.

Thrombosis

Newer views on the hemostatic derangements in liver disease have found the balance is often tipped toward a prothrombotic tendency, rather than a state of anticoagulation.[4,31] This may explain the reason that patients with acute and chronic liver disease develop clinically significant thrombosis. Retrospective studies have shown that patients with liver disease develop deep venous thrombosis (DVT) and/or pulmonary embolism (PE) with an incidence of 0.5% to 8.2%.[32] The incidence of portal vein thrombosis (PVT) in patients with cirrhosis is correlated with severity of liver disease. Patients with compensated cirrhosis have an estimated incidence of PVT of 1% and patients who are being evaluated for liver transplantation have an incidence of approximately 8% to 25%.[33,34] Initial reports implicated the development of PVT with subsequent worsening of the underlying liver disease. A recent prospective evaluation of 1243 patients with cirrhosis yielded a PVT incidence of 11%, but the development of PVT was not associated with subsequent disease progression.[35] Recognizing that patients with liver disease may have a thrombotic predilection may alter the general approach to managing these patients. Many investigators have looked for the presence of risk factors associated with peripheral and portal thrombosis, and these studies have implicated age, gender, comorbidities, nutritional status, and the presence of indwelling central lines.[36,37] One consistent factor identified in several studies was low albumin level, with one study showing 5 times greater risk of venous thromboembolism (VTE) when albumin was less than 1.9 mg/dL when compared with patients with normal albumin levels.[38–41] The INR level was not correlated with or protective against VTE.[38,42] Further studies will help elucidate which factors pose the greatest risk to thrombosis in this population.

MANAGEMENT
Antithrombotic Prophylaxis

Due to their increased risk for DVT, patients with cirrhosis should be considered for prophylaxis despite elevations in traditional markers of anticoagulation. Despite this risk, there are no specific guidelines providing recommendations regarding the prophylaxis of VTE in patients with cirrhosis.[43] There are no studies that show a clear benefit to low molecular weight heparin (LMWH), unfractionated heparin, or mechanical prophylaxis in this specific patient population. Providers can use their discretion regarding medication preference, keeping in mind complicating conditions, such as renal failure. In patients with significant thrombocytopenia (<50 K/µL), some investigators recommend holding pharmacologic prophylaxis in favor of mechanical prophylaxis with sequential compression devices.[43] It should be noted that this recommendation is based on opinion and not evidence; guidelines from the American College of Chest Physicians (ACCP) do not comment on a level below which pharmacologic prophylaxis should be held.[44]

Bleeding

Despite years of empirically treating patients with liver disease who present with hemorrhagic complications, no evidence-based guidelines or consensus recommendations have been developed to manage the hemostatic abnormalities of acute and chronic liver disease. This stems from difficulties diagnosing the coagulopathy of liver disease. As a result, there is widespread practice variation in the use of blood products in patients with liver disease. Approximately half of respondents to an informal survey at a liver disease–focused symposium consisting of hepatologists, hematologists, radiologists, surgeons, and critical care practitioners stated they would use prophylactic FFP for a liver biopsy in a patient with an INR greater than 1.5. Confusingly, more than half of the same group believed INR was not a good predictor of risk of bleeding. There was likewise a divergence in the threshold level of platelets before liver biopsy within the range of 25,000 to 50,000.[16] Experts in liver transplantation vary in the manner in which they treat coagulation abnormalities before surgery. Some universally resuscitate with FFP and platelets, whereas others argue for the use of prothrombin complex concentrate (PCC) and fibrinogen concentrates.[45,46] The lack of standardized tests has prevented rigorous prospective trials from being conducted, and although viscoelastic testing provides promise for a more standardized approach to treating patients with liver disease and hemorrhage, it is not universally available at all hospitals.

In the absence of liver disease–specific guidelines, a reasonable approach may be taken from some of the knowledge gained from in vivo and in vitro studies of the coagulation system in patients with liver disease. A main decision point comes when choosing to perform an invasive procedure on patients with abnormal values on traditional measures of the coagulation system, like platelets and INR. As mentioned previously, there has not been any evidence that INR level predicts bleeding in a number of invasive procedures. The American Association for the Study of Liver Diseases (AASLD) makes the recommendation that platelet transfusions should be considered when counts are less than 50,000 to 60,000 in patients undergoing liver biopsy.[47] This recommendation is backed by laboratory-based studies that have demonstrated platelet counts having the greatest impact on TEG-assessed clot strength.[18] Earlier studies noted platelet transfusion was the lone blood product replacement that reversed coagulation abnormalities on TEG.[48] In the clinical setting, a small series of patients with coagulation abnormalities had an increased risk of bleeding during liver biopsy when the platelet count was less than 60 K/μL.[49] Although there is evidence suggesting benefit to platelet transfusion before liver biopsy, evidence is lacking for other invasive procedures.

There is emerging evidence for the use of antifibrinolytic therapy in patients who develop bleeding. A Cochrane review has found benefit in use of tranexamic acid (TXA) in upper gastrointestinal bleeding.[50] Similarly, a meta-analysis of randomized controlled trials found the use of TXA in liver transplantation to be safe and effective.[51] With little risk and the potential for benefit, the use of TXA in patients with liver disease and clinically significant bleeding, antifibrinolytics should be considered.

The coagulation factor concentrates for reversal of vitamin K antagonist bleeding has garnered interest in their potential role for the coagulopathy of liver disease. Three-factor PCCs contain FII, FIX, FX, and FVII is present in 4-factor PCCs only. PCCs are not approved for use in patients with liver disease, but they are actively being studied in patients with ALF who are to have their coagulation abnormalities addressed immediately before liver transplantation.[52]

Thrombosis

Treatment of thrombosis is difficult in patients with liver disease due to the tenuous rebalanced state of the coagulation system and the fear of inducing or promoting bleeding events. There are no guidelines for the treatment of DVT or PE in patients with liver disease, so the safety of anticoagulation in these patients is extrapolated from the treatment of patients with PVT. Early anticoagulation of PVT represents a therapeutic consideration ever since retrospective studies found excellent recanalization rates in patients kept on anticoagulation.[53] Because of the lack of well-designed prospective trials, the AASLD does not make a recommendation for or against anticoagulation in patients with PVT and cirrhosis.[54] The ACCP does recommend anticoagulation for patients with PVT, but does not make a specific distinction regarding treating patients with concomitant PVT and cirrhosis, which differs from the AASLD guidelines.[55] The safety of anticoagulation has been examined in a few trials. The use of LMWH for treatment of 28 cases of PVT was not associated with any bleeding during 6 months of therapy.[56] In a study of 55 patients receiving both LMWH and vitamin K antagonists (VKA) for PVT, there were 5 clinical bleeding events related to anticoagulation in 19 months of follow-up. An assessment of increased bleeding risk was conducted, and was found to be statistically significant in patients with platelet counts below 50 and nonstatistically associated with use of VKA.[57]

Based on individual risks and potential benefits of therapy, the treating physician should decide on using anticoagulation for DVT, PE, and PVT. If the decision is made to prescribe anticoagulation, use of enoxaparin should be considered given greater difficulty of dosing VKAs due to the preexisting abnormalities in the INR. Patients should have appropriate screening for esophageal varices and prophylaxis with banding or nonselective beta-blockers, as this was performed in the trials that demonstrated the safety of anticoagulation in PVT.[56,57] Enoxaparin can be used at either doses of 1 mg/kg subcutaneously every 12 hours or 1.5 mg/kg daily.[58]

SUMMARY

In essence, patients with liver disease, acute and/or chronic, have a tenuous rebalanced hemostasis that is easily perturbed by various disease states. Clinicians may consider using viscoelastic testing, if available, to better assess coagulation balance to assist with clinical decisions with regard to the assessment of bleeding risk before invasive procedures. Optimizing platelet counts by transfusion and avoiding unnecessary plasma transfusion is recommended by the authors. A high INR does not convey bleeding risk in these patients, as such targeting normal levels puts the patients at risk of transfusion-associated complications without a clear benefit. Thrombotic events cause significant morbidity in patients with liver disease and treatment with anticoagulants should be considered on a case-by-case basis. Robust clinical trials are needed to address unanswered questions.

REFERENCES

1. Lisman T, Porte RJ. Rebalanced hemostasis in patients with liver disease: evidence and clinical consequences. Blood 2010;116:878–85.

2. Tripodi A, Salerno F, Chantarangkul V, et al. Evidence of normal thrombin generation in cirrhosis despite abnormal conventional coagulation tests. Hepatology 2005;41:553–8.

3. Tripodi A, Primignani M, Chantarangkul V, et al. Thrombin generation in patients with cirrhosis: the role of platelets. Hepatology 2006;44:440–5.

4. Tripodi A, Primignani M, Chantarangkul V, et al. An imbalance of pro- vs. anticoagulation factors in plasma from patients with cirrhosis. Gastroenterology 2009;137:2105–11.

5. Hollestelle MJ, Geertzen HG, Straatsberg IH, et al. Factor VIII expression in liver disease. Thromb Haemost 2004;91:267–75.

6. Dultz G, Kronenberger B, Azizi A, et al. Portal vein thrombosis as complication of romiplostim treatment in a cirrhotic patient with hepatitis C-associated immune thrombocytopenic purpura. J Hepatol 2011;55:229–32.

7. Afdhal NH, Giannini EG, Tayyab G, et al. Eltrombopag before procedures in patients with cirrhosis and thrombocytopenia. N Engl J Med 2012;367:716–24.

8. Thomas DP, Ream VJ, Stuart PK. Platelet aggregation in patients with Laennac's cirrhosis of the liver. N Engl J Med 1967;276:1344–8.

9. Violi F, Leo R, Vezza E, et al. Bleeding time in patients with cirrhosis: relation with degree of liver failure and clotting abnormalities. C.A.L.C. group. Coagulation abnormalities in cirrhosis study group. J Hepatol 1994;20:531–6.

10. Mannucci PM, Canciani MT, Forza I, et al. Changes in health and disease of the metalloprotease that cleaves von Willebrand factor. Blood 2001;98:2730–5.

11. Lisman T, Bongers TN, Adelmeijer J, et al. Elevated levels of von Willebrand factor in cirrhosis support platelet adhesion despite reduced functional capacity. Hepatology 2006;44:53–61.

12. Goodpasture EW. Fibrinolysis in chronic hepatic insufficiency. Bull Johns Hopkins Hosp 1914;25:330–2.

13. Colucci M, Binetti BM, Branca MG, et al. Deficiency of thrombin activatable fibrinolysis inhibitor in cirrhosis is associated with increased plasma fibrinolysis. Hepatology 2003;38:230–7.

14. Papatheodoridis GV, Patch D, Webster GJM, et al. Infection and hemostasis in decompensated cirrhosis: a prospective study using thromboelastography. Hepatology 1999;29:1085–90.

15. Lisman T, Bakhtari K, Adelmeijer J, et al. Intact thrombin generation and decreased fibrinolytic capacity in patients with acute liver injury or acute liver failure. J Thromb Haemost 2012;10:1312–9.

16. Caldwell SH, Hoffman M, Lisman T, et al. Coagulation disorders and hemostasis in liver disease: pathophysiology and critical assessment of current management. Hepatology 2006;44:1039–46.

17. Kang YG, Martin DJ, Marquez J, et al. Intraoperative changes in blood coagulation and thromboelastographic monitoring in liver transplantation. Anesth Analg 1985;64:888–96.

18. Stravitz RT, Lisman T, Luketic VA, et al. Minimal effects of acute liver injury/acute liver failure on hemostasis as assessed by thromboelastography. J Hepatol 2012; 56:129–36.

19. Stravitz RT. Potential applications of thromboelastography in patients with acute and chronic liver disease. Gastroenterol Hepatol (N Y) 2012;8:513–20.

20. Tripodi A, Primignani M, Chantarangkul V, et al. The coagulopathy of cirrhosis assessed by thromboelastometry and its correlation with conventional coagulation parameters. Thromb Res 2009;124:132–6.

21. Chau TN, Chan YW, Patch D, et al. Thromboelastographic changes and early rebleeding in cirrhotic patients with variceal bleeding. Gut 1998;43:267–71.

22. Sharara AI, Rockey DC. Gastroesophageal variceal hemorrhage. N Engl J Med 2001;345:669–81.

23. Shah NL, Northup PG, Caldwell SH. A clinical survey of bleeding, thrombosis, and blood product use in decompensated cirrhosis patients. Ann Hepatol 2012;11:686.

24. Ewe K. Bleeding after liver biopsy does not correlate with indices of peripheral coagulation. Dig Dis Sci 1981;26:388.

25. Gilmore IT, Burroughs A, Murray-Lyon IM, et al. Indications, methods and outcomes of percutaneous liver biopsy in England and Wales: an audit by the British

Society of Gastroenterology and the Royal College of Physicians of London. Gut 1995;36:437–41.

26. Denzer U, Helmreich-Becker I, Galle PR, et al. Liver assessment and biopsy in patients with marked coagulopathy: value of mini-laparoscopy and control of bleeding. Am J Gastroenterol 2003;98:893–900.

27. Segal JB, Dzik WH, Transfusion Medicine/Hemostasis Clinical Trials Network. Paucity of studies to support that abnormal coagulation test results predict bleeding in the setting of invasive procedures: an evidence-based review. Transfusion 2005;45:1413–25.

28. Grabau CM, Crago SF, Hoff LK, et al. Performance standards for therapeutic abdominal paracentesis. Hepatology 2004;40:484–8.

29. Townsend JC, Heard R, Powers ER, et al. Usefulness of international normalized ratio to predict bleeding complications in patients with end-stage liver disease who undergo cardiac catheterization. Am J Cardiol 2012;110:1062–5.

30. Joist JH. AICF and DIC in liver cirrhosis: expressions of a hypercoagulable state. Am J Gastroenterol 1999;94(10):2801–3.

31. Tripodi A, Primignani M, Lemma L, et al. Detection of the imbalance of procoagulant versus anticoagulant factors in cirrhosis by a simple laboratory method. Hepatology 2010;52:249–55.

32. Kolisak LP, Maynor L. Pharmacologic prophylaxis against venous thromboembolism in hospitalized patients with cirrhosis and associated coagulopathies. Am J Health Syst Pharm 2012;69:658–63.

33. Okuda K, Ohnishi K, Kimura K, et al. Incidence of portal vein thrombosis in liver cirrhosis. An angiographic study in 708 patients. Gastroenterology 1985;89(2): 279–86.

34. Francoz C, Belghiti J, Vilgrain V, et al. Splanchnic vein thrombosis in candidates for liver transplantation: usefulness of screening and anticoagulation. Gut 2005; 54:691–7.

35. Nery F, Chevret S, Condat B, et al. Causes and consequences of portal vein thrombosis in 1,243 patients with cirrhosis: results of a longitudinal study. Hepatology 2015;61:660–7.

36. Sogaard KK, Horvath-Puho E, Grobaek H, et al. Risk of venous thromboembolism in patients with liver disease: a nationwide population-based case-control study. Am J Gastroenterol 2009;104:96–101.

37. Ali M, Ananthakrishnan AN, McGinley EL, et al. Deep venous thrombosis and pulmonary embolism in hospitalized patients with cirrhosis: a nationwide analysis. Dig Dis Sci 2011;52:2152–9.

38. Northup PG, McMahon MM, Ruhl AP, et al. Coagulopathy does not fully protect hospitalized cirrhosis patients from peripheral venous thromboembolism. Am J Gastroenterol 2006;101:1524–8.

39. Gulley D, Teal E, Suvannasankha A, et al. Deep venous thrombosis and pulmonary embolism in cirrhosis patients. Dig Dis Sci 2008;53:3012–7.

40. Walsh KA, Lewis DA, Clifford TM, et al. Risk factors for venous thromboembolism in patients with chronic liver disease. Ann Pharmacother 2013;47(3):333–9.

41. Lizarraga WA, Dalia S, Reinert SE, et al. Venous thrombosis in patients with chronic liver disease. Blood Coagul Fibrinolysis 2010;21:431–5.

42. Dabbagh O, Oza A, Prakash S, et al. Coagulopathy does not protect against venous thromboembolism in hospitalized patients with chronic liver disease. Chest 2010;137:1145–9.

43. Afdhal N, McHutchinson J, Brown R, et al. Thrombocytopenia associated with chronic liver disease. J Hepatol 2008;48(6):1000–7.

44. Kahn SR, Lim W, Dunn AS, et al. Prevention of VTE in nonsurgical patients: antithrombotic therapy and prevention of thrombosis, 9th ed: American College of Chest Physicians Evidence-Based Clinical Practice Guidelines. Chest 2012; 141:e195S–226S.
45. Stanworth SJ. The evidence-based use of FFP and cryoprecipitate for abnormalities of coagulation tests and coagulopathy. Hematology Am Soc Hematol Educ Program 2007;179–86.
46. Kirchner C, Goerlinger K, Dirkmann D, et al. Safety and efficacy of prothrombin complex and fibrinogen concentrates in liver transplantation. Liver Transplant 2012;18:S189.
47. Rockey DC, Caldwell SH, Goodman ZD, et al. Liver biopsy. Hepatology 2009;49: 1017–44.
48. Clayton DG, Miro AM, Kramer DJ, et al. Quantification of thromboelastographic changes after blood component transfusion in patients with liver disease in the intensive care unit. Anesth Analg 1995;81:272–8.
49. Sharma P, McDonald GB, Banaji M. The risk of bleeding after percutaneous liver biopsy: relation to platelet count. J Clin Gastroenterol 1982;4:451–3.
50. Bennett C, Klingenberg S, Langholz E, et al. Tranexamic acid for upper gastrointestinal bleeding. Cochrane Database Syst Rev 2014;(11):CD006640.
51. Molenaar IQ, Warnaar N, Groen H, et al. Efficacy and safety of antifibrinolytic drugs in liver transplantation: a systematic review and meta-analysis. Am J Transplant 2007;7:185–94.
52. Arshad F, Ickx B, van Beem RT, et al. Prothrombin complex concentrate in the reduction of blood loss during orthotropic liver transplantation: PROTON-trial. BMC Surg 2013;13:1–12.
53. Condat B, Pessione F, Denninger MH, et al. Recent portal or mesenteric thrombosis: increased recognition and frequent recanalization on anticoagulation therapy. Hepatology 2000;32:466–70.
54. DeLeve LD, Valla DC, Garcia-Tsao G, et al. Vascular disorders of the liver. Hepatology 2009;49:1729–64.
55. Kearon C, Akl EA, Comerota AJ, et al. Antithrombotic therapy for VTE disease: antithrombotic therapy and prevention of thrombosis, 9th ed: American College of Chest Physicians Evidence-Based Clinical Practice Guidelines. Chest 2012; 141(2 Suppl):e419S–94S.
56. Amitrano L, Guardascione MA, Menchise A, et al. Safety and efficacy of anticoagulation therapy with low molecular weight heparin for portal vein thrombosis in patients with liver cirrhosis. J Clin Gastroenterol 2010;44:448–51.
57. Delgado MG, Seijo S, Yepes I, et al. Efficacy and safety of anticoagulation on patients with cirrhosis and portal vein thrombosis. Clin Gastroenterol Hepatol 2012; 10:776–83.
58. Cui SB, Shu RH, Yan SP, et al. Efficacy and safety of anticoagulation therapy with different doses of enoxaparin for portal vein thrombosis in cirrhotic patients with hepatitis B. Eur J Gastroenterol Hepatol 2015;27:914–9.

Pharmacologic Issues in Liver Disease

Jolie Gallagher, PharmD[a,b], Annie N. Biesboer, PharmD, BCPS[c],
Alley J. Killian, PharmD, BCPS[a,*]

KEYWORDS

- Pharmacology • Liver disease • Drug dosing • Pharmacokinetics • Critical illness

KEY POINTS

- The liver is a major site for drug metabolism and clearance, and any changes in liver function can subsequently affect drug disposition.
- Very few medications have recommendations for dose adjustments in liver dysfunction; however, most available recommendations are based on severity of liver disease assessed by Child-Pugh score.
- Most pharmacokinetic studies are in patients with end-stage liver disease (ESLD) with almost none in patients with acute liver failure. Dose adjustment recommendations for these patients are extrapolated from ESLD data.
- Concomitant renal dysfunction is common in patients with ESLD, so dose adjustments based on renal function should also be considered.

INTRODUCTION

The liver plays a vital role in drug disposition because it is a major site for drug metabolism and clearance; consequently, alterations in liver function cause alterations in drug disposition. However, there are no endogenous markers of hepatic clearance and traditional scoring systems such as the Child-Pugh classification (**Table 1**) do not correlate well with hepatic clearance and drug metabolism in liver disease.[1] Thus, the effect of liver dysfunction on drug disposition may be hard to determine. However, there are known changes in pharmacokinetics that occur in liver disease, particularly end-stage liver disease (ESLD), that can aide clinicians in drug dosing, and these are reviewed in this article. In addition, there are pharmacokinetic data

---

Disclosures: Authors have no disclosures.
[a] Department of Pharmaceutical Services, Emory University Hospital, 1364 Clifton Road, Northeast, Atlanta, GA 30322, USA; [b] Mercer University College of Pharmacy, Atlanta, GA; [c] Concordia University of Wisconsin School of Pharmacy, 12800 North Lake Shore Drive, Mequon, WI 53097, USA
* Corresponding author.
E-mail address: alley.killian@emoryhealthcare.org

Crit Care Clin 32 (2016) 397–410
http://dx.doi.org/10.1016/j.ccc.2016.02.003
0749-0704/16/$ – see front matter © 2016 Elsevier Inc. All rights reserved.

Table 1
Child-Pugh score

Clinical and Laboratory Criteria	Points		
	1	2	3
Ascites	None	Slight	Moderate to severe
Hepatic encephalopathy	None	Grade 1–2	Grade 3–4
Bilirubin (mg/dL)	<2	2–3	>3
Albumin (g/dL)	>3.5	2.8–3.5	<2.8
Prothrombin Time			
Time prolonged (s)	<4	4–6	>6
INR	<1.7	1.7–2.3	>2.3

Points	Grade	Description
5–6	A	Mild; well compensated
7–9	B	Moderate; significant functional compromise
10–15	C	Severe; decompensated disease

Abbreviation: INR, International Normalized Ratio.

available for select medications that are also included. Unless otherwise noted, recommendations included here are for both ESLD and acute liver failure (ALF).

PHARMACOKINETIC AND PHARMACODYNAMIC ALTERATIONS
Absorption

Little is known about the changes in the absorption of orally administered medications in patients with liver dysfunction and how these affect drug dosing. However, delayed gastric emptying can be present in patients with cirrhosis, which delays the absorption of medications by the small intestine.[2,3] Although delayed absorption of medications can occur, it does not seem to affect the extent of absorption.[3] In addition, the bioavailability of orally administered medications can be significantly increased in patients with liver dysfunction because of a reduction in first-pass metabolism. First-pass metabolism refers to the metabolism of an orally administered medication after absorption and before distribution into the systemic circulation.[2,4] The liver plays a large role in first-pass metabolism because the small intestine, where most orally administered medications are absorbed, empties into the hepatic portal circulation.[5] First-pass metabolism is avoided when medications are administered intravenously. The effect of liver dysfunction on first-pass metabolism is discussed in detail later.

Distribution

Often, patients with cirrhosis experience fluid retention and/or ascites causing an increase in volume of distribution (Vd). This increase in volume mainly affects medications that are water soluble, or hydrophilic, because they reside in serum.[2] Consequently, the dose of hydrophilic medications may need to be increased to achieve therapeutic efficacy.[3] Medications that are bound to plasma proteins can have an increased free plasma concentration in chronic liver disease. This process is multifactorial, including a reduction in the synthesis of plasma proteins, namely albumin and α_1-acid glycoprotein, as well as an increase in substances that can displace protein-bound medications, such as bilirubin.[6] Therapeutic drug monitoring of drugs that are highly protein bound should be considered, particularly for medications with a narrow therapeutic index.

Metabolism/Elimination

There are several factors that influence the liver's ability to metabolize and eliminate medications, including intrinsic drug clearance, hepatic blood flow, and the drug extraction ratio.[1,2,6] Intrinsic drug clearance refers to the ability of the liver to enzymatically metabolize a specific medication, either through phase I (eg, oxidation) or phase II (eg, glucuronidation) metabolic reactions. Phase I metabolism is performed by numerous different enzymes belonging to the cytochrome P (CYP) 450 family and seems to be affected by liver dysfunction to a much greater extent than phase II metabolism.[7] The delivery of medications to the liver relies heavily on hepatic blood flow, which can be dramatically decreased in liver dysfunction, particularly ESLD. Hepatic blood flow can be diminished further by portosystemic shunting.

The drug extraction ratio is determined by intrinsic drug clearance and hepatic blood flow and refers to the ability of the liver to metabolize and eliminate a particular medication. Details of the effect of liver disease are provided in **Table 2**.

The elimination of medications through other routes can also be decreased in patients with liver dysfunction. There is a high incidence of renal dysfunction in patients with liver dysfunction, which can prolong the activity of medications that are renally excreted. Calculation of creatinine clearance and change in the dosing regimen should be performed if necessary. Furthermore, cholestasis can lead to a decrease in the biliary excretion of some medications.

NEUROLOGY

There are several classes of neurologic medications that need careful consideration when used in critically ill patients with liver dysfunction, including antiepileptic drugs (AEDs), analgesics, and sedatives.

Antiepileptics

Most AEDs are hepatically metabolized to some extent; the presence of liver dysfunction can cause significant alterations in the pharmacokinetics of these medications. Phenytoin is a highly protein-bound, low-extraction-ratio AED that is metabolized predominately by CYP2C9 to an inactive metabolite.[8,9] The use of phenytoin in liver dysfunction may be associated with decreased elimination, therefore monitoring of free phenytoin levels is highly recommended. Lacosamide, a new AED that has low protein binding and a low extraction ratio, is excreted ~30% unchanged in the urine and undergoes CYP2C9, CYP2C19, and CYP3A4 metabolism.[9] Lacosamide was found to have a 50% to 60% increase in concentration in patients with moderate liver dysfunction (Child-Pugh B) so a maximum dose of 300 mg/d is recommended in patients with mild to moderate hepatic impairment.[8,9] There are no pharmacokinetic studies of lacosamide in severe liver dysfunction. Levetiracetam is also an AED with low protein binding and a low extraction ratio. Approximately 66% is excreted unchanged by the kidneys, whereas 24% is metabolized via hydrolysis of the acetamide group.[10] A single-dose study in patients with moderate to severe cirrhosis (Child-Pugh A, B, or C) found that patients with severe cirrhosis (Child-Pugh C) had a 57% reduction in clearance of levetiracetam; however, this group of patients also had a significantly lower creatinine clearance compared with the other groups.[10] At present there are no recommendations for dose reductions of levetiracetam in liver dysfunction but dose adjustments should be made in patients with concomitant kidney dysfunction.

Table 2
Effect of liver disease on metabolism of medications with different extraction ratios

Extraction Ratio	Bioavailability	Effect of Liver Dysfunction	Pathophysiology	Medications[a]	Dose Adjustment[b]
High (>60%)	≤40%	↑ Bioavailability	↓ Hepatic blood flow + portosystemic shunting → ↓ drug delivery to the liver	Labetalol Metoprolol Morphine Nicardipine Promethazine Sertraline Venlafaxine	Consider ↓ initial and maintenance dose
Intermediate (30%–60%)	40%–70%	↓ Hepatic clearance	↓ Enzymatic activity	Amiodarone Amitriptyline Atorvastatin Carvedilol Ciprofloxacin Codeine Diltiazem Nifedipine Haloperidol Itraconazole Mirtazapine Olanzapine Omeprazole Paroxetine Pravastatin Ranitidine Simvastatin	Consider ↓ maintenance dose

| Low (<30%) + high protein binding (≥90%) | ≥70% | ↑/↔ Hepatic clearance | ↑ Free fraction, more drug available for metabolism | Diazepam
Lansoprazole
Lorazepam
Methadone
Phenytoin
Rifampin
Trazodone
Valproic acid
Zolpidem | Therapeutic drug monitoring if narrow therapeutic index |
| Low (<30%) + low protein binding (<90%) | ≥70% | ↓ Hepatic clearance | ↓ Enzymatic activity | Acetaminophen
Alprazolam
Levetiracetam
Methylprednisolone
Metoclopramide
Metronidazole
Phenobarbital
Prednisone
Risperidone | Consider ↓ maintenance dose |

a List is not all-inclusive.
b Recommendation for orally administered medications.

Analgesics

The use of acetaminophen in patients with liver dysfunction is generally avoided, likely because of its association with hepatotoxicity. Available studies have shown that short-term, therapeutic doses (≤ 4 g/d) of acetaminophen in patients with nonalcoholic cirrhosis do not lead to accumulation or significant changes in liver function tests.[11,12] Patients with alcoholic cirrhosis may be particularly vulnerable to hepatotoxicity secondary to acetaminophen because of induction of the enzyme responsible for production of N-acetyl p-benzoquinone imine (NAPQI), a hepatotoxic metabolite, and deceased levels of glutathione, which neutralizes NAPQI. Acetaminophen use in alcoholic patients with cirrhosis should be minimized (<2 g/d) or avoided if possible. Opioids in patients with liver dysfunction should be used cautiously because they can cause sedation and precipitate hepatic encephalopathy.[12,13] Morphine, a high-extraction-ratio opioid, is metabolized by the liver to an active metabolite as well as other inactive metabolites. Many studies have shown an increased half-life and bioavailability of morphine in patients with liver dysfunction.[11,14] If used, the dosing interval should be increased and the dose of oral morphine decreased. Similarly, hydromorphone is a high-extraction-ratio opioid that has increased bioavailability in liver dysfunction; however, the half-life does not seem to be affected.[11] Both morphine and hydromorphone have neuroexcitatory metabolites that can accumulate in renal dysfunction, so avoidance in patients with concomitant renal dysfunction is recommended. Fentanyl may be preferred in patients with liver dysfunction because its pharmacokinetics seem to be largely unaffected in these patients.[14]

Sedatives

Lorazepam and midazolam are frequently used benzodiazepines for both sedation and seizure termination in the critically ill, and both are metabolized by liver. The clearance of lorazepam and midazolam is decreased in liver dysfunction, which can result in prolonged sedation.[15] In addition, midazolam has an active metabolite that is renally eliminated so the use of midazolam in patients with both liver and kidney impairment can further prolong sedation. Dexmedetomidine, an alpha-2 agonist, is another frequently used sedative in critically ill patients that is metabolized by the liver. In patients with severe hepatic dysfunction, the clearance of dexmedetomidine is impaired, which can lead to delayed emergence from sedation.[15,16]

CARDIOVASCULAR
Vasopressors

Patients with cirrhosis have a low systemic vascular resistance, increased cardiac output, and low mean arterial pressure at baseline. These hemodynamic manifestations are enhanced in the setting of critical illness and especially sepsis. Vasopressors are frequently required to maintain adequate perfusion. Norepinephrine is considered the vasopressor of choice for distributive shock in patients with cirrhosis because its stimulation of both alpha and beta receptors increases mean arterial pressure because of vasoconstrictive effects while preserving cardiac output with little increase in stroke volume compared with dopamine. There are no dosing recommendations specific to patients with liver disease and vasopressors can be titrated to patient-specific hemodynamic goals. Dopamine should generally be avoided because it can cause vasodilation of the splanchnic circulation, thereby worsening portal hypertension.[17]

β-Blockers

β-Adrenoreceptor antagonists are used in the critical care setting for a variety of indications, including hypertension and arrhythmias. Metoprolol is a commonly used selective β-adrenoreceptor antagonist that is metabolized by the liver via several different metabolic pathways.[18] It is a high-extraction-ratio medication so bioavailability is increased in liver disease (from 50% in normal subjects to 80% in cirrhosis). In addition, the area under the curve was markedly increased and the elimination half-life was prolonged following both oral and intravenous doses.[19] Dose reduction by a factor of 2 to 3 has been recommended.[18]

Antiarrhythmics

Most antiarrhythmics are metabolized by the liver and have a narrow therapeutic index, making dose adjustments clinically significant in this patient population. The most commonly used antiarrhythmics in the noncardiac critical care setting are discussed here, such as those used for atrial fibrillation. Amiodarone is likely the most commonly used antiarrhythmic in most noncardiac intensive care units (ICUs). It is extensively metabolized by the liver and has a very long half-life in patients without liver disease after prolonged oral administration (25–53 days).[20,21] Although there are no data specific to amiodarone in liver disease, it can be assumed that metabolism would be affected, resulting in an even longer half-life.[18] Diltiazem, a class IV antiarrhythmic used for rate control in atrial fibrillation, is also extensively metabolized by the liver, resulting in decreased clearance in patients with liver dysfunction. A small study of long-term oral administration in cirrhosis showed a slightly prolonged half-life and increased area under the curve of diltiazem and an active metabolite.[22] An empiric dose reduction by a factor of 2 has been suggested.[18]

QT interval prolongation is frequently associated with cirrhotic cardiomyopathy, which can worsen as severity of cirrhosis worsens. The prevalence of QT prolongation has been reported to be as high as 60% in patients with Child-Pugh grade C cirrhosis.[23] Therefore, evaluation of the baseline QT interval and continued monitoring is vital, as is assessment of medications with risk of QT prolongation.

PULMONARY

Pulmonary complications are common in ESLD.[24,25] Standard supportive-care medication therapies for dyspnea and hypoxia (eg, albuterol, inhaled steroids) can be prescribed in this patient population without need for dosing adjustments. More severe complications, such as portopulmonary hypertension, may require treatment with standard pulmonary hypertension therapies, such as synthetic prostacyclins and phosphodiesterase inhibitors.[26] There is increasing evidence supporting the use of sildenafil in this patient population.[27–29] Sildenafil undergoes metabolism via CYP3A4 and CYP2C9 to form an active metabolite. Although the manufacturer of sildenafil (Revatio) provides no dose adjustment recommendations, the manufacturer for sildenafil (Viagra) suggests a lower starting dose; therefore, it may be pertinent to be cautious with aggressive dosing of this agent in patients with ESLD.[30,31]

GASTROINTESTINAL
Acid Suppression

Proton pump inhibitors (PPIs) and histamine H2-receptor antagonists (H2RAs) are commonly prescribed agents for hospitalized patients with ESLD. These agents are generally prescribed for one of 2 indications: stress ulcer prophylaxis or treatment of gastrointestinal hemorrhages.

There is no evidence to date to recommend one PPI instead of another for any indication. However, pharmacokinetic alterations caused by hepatic impairment may warrant the selection of one agent instead of the others. Most PPIs undergo significant metabolism via the CYP system. Decreased clearance of these agents has been documented in the literature, suggesting that lower dosages of these agents may be appropriate in this patient population.[7] Esomeprazole manufacturer recommendations suggest a maximum dose of 20 mg daily in patients with severe hepatic impairment.[32] Omeprazole and lansoprazole manufacturers do not provide specific dose adjustment recommendations, but it may be appropriate to suggest dose reductions in patients with severe liver impairment given documentation of decreased clearance. In contrast, current literature supports limited effect of hepatic impairment, regardless of severity, on the pharmacokinetics of pantoprazole.[33] No dose adjustment is currently suggested for this particular agent, and it may be the most favorable agent for use in this patient population.

With regard to H2RAs, famotidine seems to have a more favorable pharmacokinetic profile in this patient population than ranitidine. In one pharmacokinetic evaluation of famotidine use in the population of patients with ESLD, famotidine clearance was noted to be reduced in patients with decompensated liver disease, but the investigators concluded that this was likely related to concomitant impaired renal function and unlikely to be directly related to impaired liver function.[34] Ranitidine has documented increased neuropsychiatric complications in patients with ESLD and should likely be avoided in this patient population.[35]

Antiemetics

Nausea, vomiting, and decreased gastrointestinal motility are also common complications associated with ESLD and ALF. Metoclopramide is a commonly used agent given its promotility and antiemetic effects. However, metoclopramide is subject to first-pass metabolism, has significant plasma protein binding properties, and undergoes significant hepatic metabolism so dose reductions should be considered in patients with ESLD.[36,37] Also, metoclopramide is renally excreted so a dose reduction is crucial in patients with concomitant renal dysfunction.[38] A 50% dose reduction is appropriate in patients with cirrhosis.[7] Similarly, ondansetron undergoes extensive first-pass metabolism, is highly protein bound, and is extensively metabolized via the CYP system. Patients with severe hepatic impairment warrant a daily dosage of 8 mg or less.[39]

Molecular Adsorbent Recirculating System

The molecular adsorbent recirculating system (MARS) is becoming a more widely used therapy in patients with severe, decompensated liver disease and ALF. Data are currently limited regarding the effects MARS has on medication clearance. Although data are limited, medications that are highly bound to albumin may be excreted via MARS and dosing modifications may need to be considered. Further research is necessary to understand the implications of the use of MARS on specific medication clearance.

RENAL

Renal dosing adjustments are required for many medications; however, these adjustments are significantly complicated by the pharmacokinetic alterations, particularly fluctuations in distribution, that occur in patients with hepatic impairment. Patients with an increased Vd secondary to ascites or critical illness potentially have a decreased renal clearance of medications given the kidney's decreased access to the medication. Also, medications that are usually protein bound typically have greater renal clearance in patients with hepatic impairment secondary to decreased protein production, and therefore a greater free concentration available for elimination by the kidney.

There is a potential for critically ill patients with hepatic impairment to require continuous renal replacement therapy (CRRT). Dose adjustments are commonly necessary for medications with specific pharmacokinetic properties such as low protein binding, small Vd, and small molecular size. It is critical to understand that these properties may be significantly altered from baseline in patients with hepatic impairment. In order to appropriately dose medications in patients with hepatic impairment receiving CRRT, critical evaluation of each medication's pharmacokinetic properties in relation to both hepatic clearance and CRRT clearance is essential.

HEMATOLOGY
Venous Thromboembolism Prophylaxis and Anticoagulation

Historically, the endogenous coagulopathy in patients with ESLD caused by decreased production of vitamin K clotting factors and platelets was thought to be protective against the development of venous thromboembolism (VTE).[40] More recent studies have called this theory of autoanticoagulation into question and shown that these patients also have decreased production of anticoagulation factors and may be at an increased or similar risk of VTE compared with hospitalized patients without ESLD.[41] Literature evaluating the safety of pharmacologic prophylaxis in ESLD is limited but does raise concern for an increased risk of bleeding complications.[42,43] In addition, evidence-based VTE prophylaxis guidelines provide no specific recommendations for patients with liver disease but advise against the use of pharmacologic prophylaxis in patients with significant bleeding risk, defined as platelet count less than 50,000/μL, liver failure, and International Normalized Ratio (INR) greater than 1.5.[44] Note that there are limited data in critically ill cirrhotic patients. A recent retrospective study of 798 patients found that the incidence of VTE in critically ill cirrhotic patients was not statistically different from that in noncirrhotic patients, although rates were low at 2.7% and 7.6%, respectively. Cirrhotic patients were less likely to receive pharmacologic prophylaxis.[45] ESLD and associated coagulopathy (increase in INR) alone should not be considered a contraindication to pharmacologic prophylaxis, although careful evaluation of risk versus benefit should be done on a patient-by-patient basis. As a result of the increased risk of VTE, anticoagulation therapy is increasingly being used in patients with ESLD. There are limited data on the safety of therapeutic anticoagulation in the hospital setting in patients with ESLD, especially in critically ill patients.

If pharmacologic prophylaxis or therapeutic anticoagulation is initiated with unfractionated heparin there are no dosing considerations specific to patients with liver dysfunction. Many of these patients have concomitant renal dysfunction and, because low-molecular-weight heparins (with the exception of dalteparin) are renally cleared, they are considered to be at higher risk for bleeding complications.

Patients with ALF frequently have an acute coagulopathy and are at high risk of bleeding complications. There are no data evaluating the use of VTE prophylaxis or therapeutic anticoagulation in this population. Mechanical prophylaxis only is typically recommended during the acute phase of the disease process.

Heparin-Induced Thrombocytopenia

Of the medications that are used for anticoagulation in the setting of heparin-induced thrombocytopenia, argatroban is the only one with pharmacologic considerations in liver dysfunction. Argatroban is a direct thrombin inhibitor that is hepatically metabolized primarily by CYP3A4/CYP3A5 to nonactive metabolites. The elimination half-life is approximately 45 minutes in healthy volunteers but is increased 3-fold in patients with moderate hepatic impairment (Child-Pugh score >6) along with a 4-fold decrease in systemic clearance. Furthermore, anticoagulant responses returned to baseline in 2 to 4 hours in healthy volunteers but took at least 6 hours (up to 20 hours) in patients with hepatic impairment.[46] As a result, the recommended starting dose of argatroban per the manufacturer is decreased from 2 μg/kg/min to 0.5 μg/kg/min in patients with moderate or severe hepatic impairment.[47] A retrospective study supporting this reduced starting dose also recommended delaying the monitoring of the activated partial thromboplastin time to at least 4 to 5 hours after initiation or dose adjustments (compared with the standard of 2 hours) because of the longer time required to achieve steady state concentrations.[48] Retrospective studies of argatroban in critically ill patients describe significantly reduced dosing requirements.[49,50] One found a 57% reduction in dose compared with non–critically ill patients and that dose requirements were inversely related to Sequential Organ Failure Assessment score.[49] The investigators of a second study recommended a starting dose of one-tenth to one-eighth of the standard starting dose. The mean argatroban dose was even lower in the critically ill patients who also had hepatic impairment compared to those without.[50]

INFECTIOUS DISEASE

Patients with both ALF and ESLD are at significant risk of various types of infection.[51–54] Infection either exists on admission or is acquired during hospitalization in approximately 25% to 30% of patients with ESLD.[51,52] As in the general ICU population, multidrug-resistant pathogens are of increasing prevalence in ESLD and should be taken into consideration when selecting antibiotics for nosocomial infections.[51] As a result of these findings, use of antimicrobials in this patient population is significant. Hepatic dysfunction affects several pharmacokinetic parameters, which affects antimicrobial dosing, including decreased protein binding, metabolism, and renal elimination. As previously mentioned, a significant portion of these patients have concomitant renal dysfunction, which affects the dosing of most antimicrobials. In contrast with the available literature to guide dosing of antimicrobials in renal dysfunction, there is a shortage of literature on the pharmacokinetics of antimicrobials in liver dysfunction. The antimicrobials used in the ICU that have specific dosing recommendations in the package labeling based on Child-Pugh score are limited to metronidazole, tigecycline, caspofungin, and voriconazole. A recently published review extensively evaluated the pharmacokinetic literature for commonly used antibiotics that undergo hepatic or mixed renal-hepatobiliary clearance. In addition to noting recommendations that exist in product labeling, the investigators made additional dose adjustment recommendations by Child-Pugh score based on the available pharmacokinetic literature. Antibiotics included that are pertinent to the ICU setting include clindamycin, metronidazole, nafcillin, quinupristin-dalfopristin, rifampin, and tigecycline.[55]

Recent literature has highlighted the inadequacy of standard antibiotic dosing regimens in the critically ill. Specifically, the ability to achieve desired concentrations is decreased, which has been associated with adverse patient outcomes.[56] Both ESLD and critical illness are well known to be associated with increased Vd.

Hydrophilic drugs, such as β-lactam antibiotics, are of concern because of the risk of decreased plasma concentrations and thus efficacy. Increased loading doses should be considered.[57]

In addition, ESLD has been reported to be a risk factor for several antibiotic-related toxicities, including β-lactam–induced neutropenia and aminoglycoside-related nephrotoxicity.[58,59]

SUMMARY

Although the liver plays a vital role in drug disposition there are few data and limited guidance for drug dosing in liver disease. Available evidence and drug dosing recommendations come from pharmacokinetic studies in patients with ESLD with virtually none in patients with ALF. Known changes in pharmacokinetic parameters in liver dysfunction can help to guide drug dosing and, if possible, therapeutic drug monitoring should be used.

REFERENCES

1. Kim JW, Phongsamran PV. Drug-induced liver disease and drug use considerations in liver disease. J Pharm Pract 2009;22:278–89.
2. Lin S, Smith BS. Drug dosing considerations for the critically ill patient with liver disease. Crit Care Nurs Clin North Am 2010;22:335–40.
3. Delco F, Tchambaz L, Schlienger R, et al. Dose adjustment in patients with liver disease. Drug Saf 2005;28:529–45.
4. Pond SM, Tozer TN. First-pass elimination. Basic concepts and clinical consequences. Clin Pharmacokinet 1984;9:1–25.
5. Pang KS. Modeling of intestinal drug absorption: roles of transporters and metabolic enzymes (for the Gillette Review Series). Drug Metab Dispos 2003;31: 1507–19.
6. Verbeeck RK, Horsmans Y. Effect of hepatic insufficiency on pharmacokinetics and drug dosing. Pharm World Sci 1998;20:183–92.
7. Rodighiero V. Effects of liver disease on pharmacokinetics. An update. Clin Pharmacokinet 1999;37:399–431.
8. Asconape JJ. Use of antiepileptic drugs in hepatic and renal disease. Handb Clin Neurol 2014;119:417–32.
9. Anderson GD, Hakimian S. Pharmacokinetic of antiepileptic drugs in patients with hepatic or renal impairment. Clin Pharmacokinet 2014;53:29–49.
10. Brockmoller J, Thomsen T, Wittstock M, et al. Pharmacokinetics of levetiracetam in patients with moderate to severe liver cirrhosis (Child-Pugh classes A, B, and C): characterization by dynamic liver function tests. Clin Pharmacol Ther 2005;77: 529–41.
11. Bosilkovska M, Walder B, Besson M, et al. Analgesics in patients with hepatic impairment: pharmacology and clinical implications. Drugs 2012;72: 1645–69.
12. Dwyer JP, Jayasekera C, Nicoll A. Analgesia for the cirrhotic patient: a literature review and recommendations. J Gastroenterol Hepatol 2014;29:1356–60.
13. Yogaratnam D, Miller MA, Smith BS. The effects of liver and renal dysfunction on the pharmacokinetics of sedatives and analgesics in the critically ill patient. Crit Care Nurs Clin North Am 2005;17:245–50.
14. Imani F, Motavaf M, Safari S, et al. The therapeutic use of analgesics in patients with liver cirrhosis: a literature review and evidence-based recommendations. Hepat Mon 2014;14:e23539.

15. Barr J, Fraser GL, Puntillo K, et al. Clinical practice guidelines for the management of pain, agitation, and delirium in adult patients in the intensive care unit. Crit Care Med 2013;41:263–306.
16. Hughes CG, McGrane S, Pandharipande PP. Sedation in the intensive care setting. Clin Pharmacol 2012;4:53–63.
17. Canabal JM, Kramer DJ. Management of sepsis in patients with liver failure. Curr Opin Crit Care 2008;14:189–97.
18. Klotz U. Antiarrhythmics: elimination and dosage considerations in hepatic impairment. Clin Pharmacokinet 2007;46:985–96.
19. Regardh CG, Jordö L, Ervik M, et al. Pharmacokinetics of metoprolol in patients with hepatic cirrhosis. Clin Pharmacokinet 1981;6:375–88.
20. Latini R, Tognoni G, Kates RE. Clinical pharmacokinetics of amiodarone. Clin Pharmacokinet 1984;9:136–56.
21. Gill J, Heel RC, Fitton A. Amiodarone. An overview of its pharmacological properties, and review of its therapeutic use in cardiac arrhythmias. Drugs 1992;43: 69–110.
22. Kurosawa S, Kurosawa N, Owada E, et al. Pharmacokinetics of diltiazem in patients with liver cirrhosis. Int J Clin Pharmacol Res 1990;10:311–8.
23. Bernardi M, Calandra S, Colantoni A, et al. Q-T interval prolongation in cirrhosis: prevalence, relationship with severity, and etiology of the disease and possible pathogenetic factors. Hepatology 1998;27:28–34.
24. Roberts DN, Arguedas MR, Fallon MB. Cost-effectiveness of screening for hepatopulmonary syndrome in liver transplant candidates. Liver Transpl 2007;13:206–14.
25. Fallon MB, Abrams GA. Pulmonary dysfunction in chronic liver disease. Hepatology 2000;32:859–65.
26. Stauber RE, Olschewski H. Portopulmonary hypertension: short review. Eur J Gastroenterol Hepatol 2010;22:385–90.
27. Shen YC, Wen FQ, Yi Q. The clinical application of sildenafil in porto pulmonary hypertension. Zhonghua Jie He Hu Xi Za Zhi 2011;34:691–3 [in Chinese].
28. Hollatz TJ, Musat A, Westphal S, et al. Treatment with sildenafil and treprostinil allows successful liver transplantation of patients with moderate to severe portopulmonary hypertension. Liver Transpl 2012;18:686–95.
29. Cadden IS, Greanya ED, Erb SR, et al. The use of sildenafil to treat portopulmonary hypertension prior to liver transplantation. Ann Hepatol 2009;8:158–61.
30. Viagra® [package insert]. New York, NY: Pfizer Labs; 2015.
31. Revatio® [package insert]. New York, NY: Pfizer Labs; 2015.
32. Nexium® [package insert]. Wilmington, DE: AstraZeneca Pharmaceuticals LP; 2014.
33. Ferron GM, Preston RA, Noveck RJ, et al. Pharmacokinetics of pantoprazole in patients with moderate and severe hepatic dysfunction. Clin Ther 2001;23:1180–92.
34. Vincon G, Baldit C, Couzigou P, et al. Pharmacokinetics of famotidine in patients with cirrhosis and ascites. Eur J Clin Pharmacol 1992;43:559–62.
35. Vial T, Goubier C, Bergeret A, et al. Side effects of ranitidine. Drug Saf 1991;6: 94–117.
36. Bernardi M, Trevisani F, Gasbarrini G. Metoclopramide administration in advanced liver disease. Gastroenterology 1986;91:523.
37. Uribe M, Ballesteros A, Strauss R, et al. Successful administration of metoclopramide for the treatment of nausea in patients with advanced liver disease. A double-blind controlled trial. Gastroenterology 1985;88:757–62.
38. Reglan® [package insert]. Baudette, MN: ANI Pharmaceuticals, Inc.; 2011.
39. Zofran® [package insert]. Research Triangle Park, NC: GlaxoSmithKline; 2014.

40. Heit JA, Silverstein MD, Mohr DN, et al. Risk factors for deep vein thrombosis and pulmonary embolism: a population-based case-control study. Arch Intern Med 2000;160:809–15.

41. Wu H, Nguyen GC. Liver cirrhosis is associated with venous thromboembolism among hospitalized patients in a nationwide US study. Clin Gastroenterol Hepatol 2010;8:800–5.

42. Reichert JA, Hlavinka PF, Stolzfus JC. Risk of hemorrhage in patients with chronic liver disease and coagulopathy receiving pharmacologic venous thromboembolism prophylaxis. Pharmacotherapy 2014;34:1043–9.

43. Shatzel J, Dulai PS, Harbin D, et al. Safety and efficacy of pharmacological thromboprophylaxis for hospitalized patients with cirrhosis: a single-center retrospective cohort study. J Thromb Haemost 2015;13:1245–53.

44. Kahn SR, Lim W, Dunn AS, et al. Prevention of VTE in nonsurgical patients: antithrombotic therapy and prevention of thrombosis, 9th ed: American College of Chest Physicians Evidence-Based Clinical Practice Guidelines. Chest 2012; 141:e195S–226S.

45. Al-Dorzi HM, Tamim HM, Aldawood AS, et al. Venous thromboembolism in critically ill cirrhotic patients: practices of prophylaxis and incidence. Thrombosis 2013;2013:807526.

46. Swan SK, Hursting MJ. The pharmacokinetics and pharmacodynamics of argatroban: effects of age, gender, and hepatic or renal dysfunction. Pharmacotherapy 2000;20:318–29.

47. Argatroban® [package insert]. Houston, TX: Encysive Pharmaceuticals, Inc; 2015.

48. Levine RL, Hursting MJ, McCollum D. Argatroban therapy in heparin-induced thrombocytopenia with hepatic dysfunction. Chest 2006;129:1167–75.

49. Keegan SP, Gallagher EM, Ernst NE, et al. Effects of critical illness and organ failure on therapeutic argatroban dosage requirements in patients with suspected or confirmed heparin-induced thrombocytopenia. Ann Pharmacother 2009;43: 19–27.

50. Saugel B, Phillip V, Moessmer G, et al. Argatroban therapy for heparin-induced thrombocytopenia in ICU patients with multiple organ dysfunction syndrome: a retrospective study. Crit Care 2010;14:R90.

51. Fernandez J, Acevedo J, Castro M, et al. Prevalence and risk factors of infections by multiresistant bacteria in cirrhosis: a prospective study. Hepatology 2012;55: 1551–61.

52. Fernandez J, Navasa M, Gómez J, et al. Bacterial infections in cirrhosis: epidemiological changes with invasive procedures and norfloxacin prophylaxis. Hepatology 2002;35:140–8.

53. Rolando N, Harvey F, Brahm J, et al. Fungal infection: a common, unrecognised complication of acute liver failure. J Hepatol 1991;12:1–9.

54. Rolando N, Harvey F, Brahm J, et al. Prospective study of bacterial infection in acute liver failure: an analysis of fifty patients. Hepatology 1990;11:49–53.

55. Halilovic J, Heintz BH. Antibiotic dosing in cirrhosis. Am J Health Syst Pharm 2014;71:1621–34.

56. Roberts JA, Paul SK, Akova M, et al. DALI: defining antibiotic levels in intensive care unit patients: are current beta-lactam antibiotic doses sufficient for critically ill patients? Clin Infect Dis 2014;58:1072–83.

57. Udy AA, Roberts JA, Lipman J. Clinical implications of antibiotic pharmacokinetic principles in the critically ill. Intensive Care Med 2013;39:2070–82.

58. Moore RD, Smith CR, Lietman PS. Increased risk of renal dysfunction due to interaction of liver disease and aminoglycosides. Am J Med 1986;80:1093–7.
59. Singh N, Yu VL, Mieles LA, et al. Beta-lactam antibiotic-induced leukopenia in severe hepatic dysfunction: risk factors and implications for dosing in patients with liver disease. Am J Med 1993;94:251–6.

Infections in Liver Disease

Rahul S. Nanchal, MD, MS[a],*, Shahryar Ahmad, MD[b]

KEYWORDS

- Infections • Cirrhosis • Sepsis • Acute on chronic liver failure • Septic shock
- Cirrhosis-associated immune dysfunction • Antibiotics • Acute kidney injury

KEY POINTS

- Infections are common in end-stage liver disease and the incidence is much higher than in the general population.
- Infectious insults are frequent precipitators of decompensated cirrhosis and acute on chronic liver failure.
- Cirrhosis is a state of systemic inflammation and immune dysfunction leading to enhanced susceptibility to infections.
- Spontaneous bacterial peritonitis and urinary tract infections are the most common infections in cirrhosis.
- The spectrum of microorganisms is shifting with the emergence of resistant organisms and this has important implications for therapy and prophylaxis.

INTRODUCTION

Infectious complications in end-stage liver disease (ESLD) are the leading cause of mortality, morbidity,[1,2] and the development of acute on chronic liver failure (ACLF). Once infection occurs, the host with cirrhosis is vulnerable to further infections and complications, such as acute kidney injury (AKI), de-listing from liver transplantation, prolonged hospital stays, and multiple organ failure. In this review, we discuss the importance of changing spectrum of infections in liver disease, new diagnostic modalities with their limitations, and current management strategies for a focused approach in treatment.

EPIDEMIOLOGY OF INFECTIONS IN LIVER DISEASE

Despite better understanding of the mechanisms of increased susceptibility to infection in chronic liver disease and advances in treatment, occurrence of infection is still

Disclosures: None.
[a] Critical Care Fellowship Program, Medical Intensive Care Unit, Division of Pulmonary and Critical Care Medicine, Medical College of Wisconsin, Suite E 5200, 9200 West Wisconsin Avenue, Milwaukee, WI 53226, USA; [b] Division of Pulmonary and Critical Care Medicine, Medical College of Wisconsin, Suite E 5200, 9200 West Wisconsin Avenue, Milwaukee, WI 53226, USA
* Corresponding author.
E-mail address: Rnanchal@mcw.edu

Crit Care Clin 32 (2016) 411–424
http://dx.doi.org/10.1016/j.ccc.2016.03.006
0749-0704/16/$ – see front matter © 2016 Elsevier Inc. All rights reserved.

associated with major morbidity and mortality. Between 25% and 35% of patients with cirrhosis either have infection at admission or acquire an infection during their hospitalization. The incidence of infections in patients with cirrhosis is 4 to 5 times greater than in the general population.

Incidence/Prevalence

According to one study, approximately 30% of bacterial infections in patients with cirrhosis were community acquired, 30% were health care associated (HCA; infections that occurred in the first 2 days of admission in patients in contact with the health care environment in the past 3 months), and 40% were nosocomial. Fernandez and colleagues[3,4] prospectively studied bacterial infections among hospitalized patients with cirrhosis and found that among 1567 admissions for decompensated cirrhosis, 507 admissions (32%) had infections on admission or during hospitalization. A follow-up study of 1578 admissions between 2005 and 2007 for complications of cirrhosis reported that 390 admissions (25%) had infections. Merli and colleagues[5] reported a prevalence of 36% in the study of 150 patients with cirrhosis, and Borzio and colleagues[6] in their prospective study of 450 patients reported a similar prevalence of 34%.

Significance of Infectious Insult in Liver Disease

It is well established that infections contribute to a high morbidity and mortality in patients with liver disease. The natural history of cirrhosis is characterized by an asymptomatic phase, referred to as "compensated cirrhosis," followed by a progressive phase marked by the development of complications of portal hypertension and/or liver dysfunction, designated "decompensated cirrhosis." Progression of the decompensated disease may be accelerated by the development of other complications, such as bleeding, renal impairment, and sepsis.[7] Arvaniti and colleagues,[8] in a large meta-analysis, found a fourfold increase in mortality for patients with cirrhosis with infection compared with similar patients with cirrhosis who were not infected.

In nonalcoholic fatty liver disease (NAFLD), progression to nonalcoholic steatohepatitis (NASH) and advanced disease has been linked to endotoxemia.[9] Impaired immune function in acute liver failure leads to an increased incidence of bacterial and fungal infections.[10,11] These infections are associated with increasing severity of complications, such as worsening hepatic encephalopathy but interestingly do not seem to adversely influence outcomes.[12,13] This may be due to increased surveillance and heightened alertness for bacterial infection as well as early (preemptive) therapy with effective antimicrobials.[14] Similarly, patients with liver failure awaiting transplantation are at increased risk of infections, and although infections before transplantation may not affect mortality, in the posttransplant period early bacterial infections are a major cause of mortality.[15,16]

Major Risk Factors of Infection in Liver Disease

Merli and colleagues[5] prospectively studied outcomes of 150 patients with cirrhosis and examined putative risk factors for infections. On multivariate analysis, a history of previous infection in the past 12 months, a model for end-stage liver disease (MELD) score of 15 or greater, and a diagnosis of protein malnutrition were independent predictors for infections and sepsis.

In other studies, prior history of gastrointestinal bleeding, high Child-Pugh scores, low albumin ascites, and prior history of spontaneous bacterial peritonitis emerged as some other risk factors associated with increased risk of infection. Further, the spectrum of infections in liver disease has gradually shifted toward the emergence of multidrug-resistant bacterial isolates. Fernandez and colleagues[4] found that nosocomial acquisition of infection, long-term norfloxacin prophylaxis, use of beta lactam antibiotics within the past 3 months, and infections with multidrug-resistant bacteria in the past 6 months before index hospitalization were independent predictors of infection by multidrug-resistant bacteria.

Types of Infection in Liver Disease

Spontaneous bacterial peritonitis (SBP) and urinary tract infections are the most frequent infections, followed by pneumonia, skin and soft tissue infections, and bacteremia.[17] Bajaj and colleagues[18] reported that second infections independently increase mortality in patients with cirrhosis. In this prospective study of 207 patients, the most common first infection at the time of admission was urinary tract infection (UTI) (25%), followed by SBP (23%), spontaneous bacteremia (21%), and skin (13%) and lower respiratory infections (8%). *Clostridium difficile* was found in 5% of patients. Most infections (71%) were HCA. Twenty-four percent of patients developed a second infection during their hospitalization. Most second infections were respiratory (28%), UTI (26%), and *C difficile* (12%). *C difficile* infections were associated with the highest case fatality rates. In another study, which included 946 patients, the most common infection reported was SBP, followed by UTI, cellulitis, pneumonia, spontaneous bacteremia, purulent bronchitis, catheter infection, secondary peritonitis, spontaneous empyema, and endocarditis.[4]

Shift of Spectrum to Resistant Infections

Most studies assessing the etiology and clinical types of bacterial infections in cirrhosis from the 1980s reported that 70% to 80% of isolated organisms were gram-negative bacteria (GNB).[3] Multidrug-resistant organisms were not reported during that time period. Chronic antibiotic prophylaxis with quinolones for SBP, change in practices including more aggressive resuscitation in intensive care units, extension of liver transplant programs, and the widespread use of invasive procedures, such as central venous catheters, have likely contributed to the change in spectrum of bacterial infections with an increase in emergence of resistant strains.

In a prospective study of infections in patients with cirrhosis, a significantly higher number of quinolone-resistant GNB and trimethoprim-sulfamethoxazole–resistant GNB were isolated in patients receiving long-term quinolone prophylaxis. Most culture-positive community-acquired infections were due to GNB; however, nosocomial infections were mainly secondary to gram-positive cocci (GPC). GNB were isolated in SBP and UTIs, whereas, in contrast, the most frequent bacterial isolates in bacteremia associated with therapeutic invasive procedures and catheter sepsis were GPC.[3]

The same group of investigators later reported 669 infections studies over 2 time periods (2005–2007 and 2010–2011). They found that multidrug-resistant infections comprised nearly 30% of cases and were associated with higher rates of septic shock, treatment failure, and poor prognosis as compared with infections caused by susceptible strains.[4] Similarly, Bajaj and colleagues,[18] in a cohort of 207 patients, reported that the first infection was caused by vancomycin-resistant enterococci in 10 isolates, methicillin-resistant *Staphylococcus aureus* in 7, fluoroquinolone-resistant GNB in 18, and extended-spectrum beta-lactamase resistance in 6 isolates; thus 20% of first infections were caused by resistant bacteria.

PATHOGENESIS OF INFECTION

Enhanced susceptibility to infection in cirrhosis is postulated to be initiated by bacterial translocation to extra-intestinal sites mediated by a combination of an alteration of the normal gut flora resulting in bacterial overgrowth, impaired host defenses, and physical damage to the intestinal mucosa (**Fig. 1**). CAID is a multifactorial state of systemic immune dysfunction that decreases the ability to clear cytokines, bacteria, and endotoxins from the circulation.[19] CAID occurrence in cirrhosis is a manifestation of two simultaneous processed - cirrhosis associated immunodeficiency and cirrhosis induced systemic inflammation.

Cirrhosis-Associated Immunodeficiency

Immune surveillance function of the liver is affected because of ongoing fibrosis and porto-systemic shunting. Cirrhosis compromises Kupffer cells and sinusoidal-endothelial cells, which comprise the reticulo-endothelial system and are strategically placed in sinusoidal vasculature to provide a major immune barrier against endotoxins and bacteria. Similarly, circulating immune cells (neutrophils, monocytes, lymphocytes) demonstrate suboptimal activity related to increased sequestration in spleen, impaired function of surface receptors, impaired phagocytic activity, and impaired memory function. These factors in concert play a pivotal role in acquired immune deficiency in liver disease.

Cirrhosis-Induced Systemic Inflammation

Persistent activation of circulating immune cells causes increased production and enhanced serum levels of proinflammatory markers as well as upregulated expression of cell activation markers. The evidence of systemic inflammation is supported by increased respiratory burst of neutrophils, upregulated expression of HLA-DR and activation/costimulatory molecules CD80 and CD 86 on monocytes, increased surface expression of activation antigens on T cells, and increased responsiveness of cells to cytokines leading to a proinflammatory state resulting in increased levels of interleukin (IL)-1, IL-6, IL-17, and tumor necrosis factor (TNF)-alpha. Pathogen-associated molecular patterns (PAMPs) from enteric bacterial organisms and damage-associated

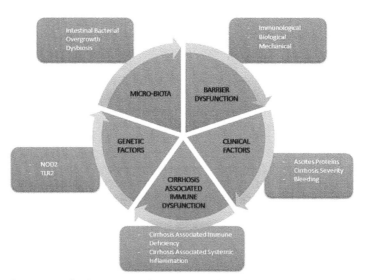

Fig. 1. Pathogenesis of infection in cirrhosis: bacterial translocation. CAID is a multifactorial state of systemic immune dysfunction that decreases the ability to clear cytokines, bacteria, and endotoxins from the circulation.[19] CAID occurrence in cirrhosis is a manifestation of two.

molecular patterns, originating from the host tissue on injury, recognize pathogen recognition receptors, expressed on innate immune cells. This leads to gene expression and increased production of proinflammatory and anti-inflammatory cytokines leading a cascade of responses driving the adaptive immune system.

The pattern of cellular activation and cytokine release varies based on the stage of liver disease. Stable compensated state of liver cirrhosis is a predominantly proinflammatory state with increased expression of activation antigens on immune cells resulting in increased serum levels of proinflammatory and anti-inflammatory cytokines. In later stages of cirrhosis, as well as ACLF, the spectrum of immune dysfunction changes from a proinflammatory state to one of immune paralysis. This immune reprogramming is thought to be secondary to decreased phagocytic activity and decreased TNF-alpha expression as seen in experimental studies of animal models. In summary, in the decompensated, ascitic stage of cirrhosis, gut bacterial translocation and PAMPs released from the leaky gut further activate the immune system and aggravate systemic inflammation. Immune response reprogramming occurs after constant endotoxin exposure and the predominantly proinflammatory cirrhosis-associated immune dysfunction (CAID) syndrome phenotype switches to an immune-deficient one of severely decompensated cirrhosis.

CHALLENGES IN THE DIAGNOSIS OF INFECTIONS IN LIVER DISEASE

In the general population, the host response to infection usually manifests as the systemic inflammatory response syndrome (SIRS). However SIRS is present in 10% to 30% of patients with decompensated cirrhosis who do not have an underlying infectious etiology. Similarly, infections in patients with cirrhosis may present without SIRS. Moreover, clinical manifestations of SIRS in cirrhosis may carry less diagnostic accuracy. For example, the use of beta blockers for portal hypertension may frequently mask tachycardia. Conversely, hepatic encephalopathy, tense ascites, hyperdynamic circulatory state, and hypersplenism, all of which are frequent manifestations of cirrhosis, may alter heart rate, respiratory rate, temperature, and white blood cell count independent of infection. Thus, the use of SIRS in cirrhosis cannot be reliably used as an indicator of infection. Further, many infections in patients with cirrhosis, particularly SBP, are frequently culture negative. Nevertheless, SIRS may still be used as a useful prognostic indicator, as its presence has been associated with higher probability of portal hypertension–related complications.[20]

Because signs and symptoms of bacterial infection might be subtle in patients with liver disease, a high clinical index of suspicion is warranted. All hospitalized patients with cirrhosis should be considered as having a potential infection unless proven otherwise.[17] Because early diagnosis is essential to instituting prompt therapy and improving outcomes, biomarkers may be helpful in the assessment of the presence of infection. C-reactive protein (CRP) and procalcitonin (PCT) are 2 such acute-phase reactants that are used as early markers of infection in the general population.[21]

A recent study reported that in decompensated cirrhosis, persistently high levels of CRP were associated with high short-term mortality.[22] Patients with liver disease may have decreased levels of CRP and PCT, because these proteins are synthesized in hepatocytes. However, the predictive value of these acute-phase reactants has been found to be similar in patients with and without cirrhosis.[23,24] Levels of these acute-phase reactants correlate with clinical course and outcome of sepsis in cirrhosis.[25] It is, however, important to note that levels of CRP can stay persistently elevated despite resolution of infection in a large percentage of patients with cirrhosis.[22] Randomized control trials have shown that PCT levels can help guide antibiotic therapy in infections; however, it has not been studied in patients specifically with liver disease.[26] Moreover, in many cases the negative predictive value of these biomarkers seems to be much more useful than their positive predictive value.

Because the development of infections in patients with cirrhosis heralds a complicated clinical course with poorer outcomes in comparison with those without infections, prognostic scoring systems are used to stratify patients at high risk of developing morbidity and mortality.

MELD has been validated as a predictor of mortality in critically ill patients with cirrhosis and performs better than some other commonly used indices in patients without cirrhosis, such as the Simplified Acute Physiology Score II (SAPS II).[27] It also may be predictive of worse outcomes in patients with cirrhosis being treated for infections. In one study, Viasus and colleagues[28] found that high MELD scores in patients with cirrhosis who developed community-acquired pneumonia were predictive of increased mortality.

Development of severe infections in patients with cirrhosis often leads to occurrence of organ failures, particularly renal failure and finally multiple organ failure. Chronic liver failure–sequential assessment of organ failure (CLIF-SOFA) score, which is a modification of the SOFA score, has been used to define the presence of specific organ system failures in patients with cirrhosis. Patients with organ failures were classified as having ACLF with 3 grades of severity. CLIF-SOFA accurately predicted mortality, with mortality increasing as the number of failing organs increased (20% 28-day mortality with 1 organ failure and 70% mortality with 3 organ failures). Although there are many precipitants of ACLF, the most common precipitant was infection.[29] Thus, extrahepatic organ failures in conjunction with clinical markers may be used to prognosticate patients with cirrhosis with severe infections.

CONSEQUENCES OF INFECTION IN LIVER DISEASE
Acute on Chronic Liver Failure

Infections are the most frequent trigger to ACLF, a syndrome in patients with chronic liver disease with or without previously diagnosed cirrhosis, which is characterized by acute hepatic decompensation resulting in liver failure (jaundice and prolongation of the International Normalized Ratio) and one or more extrahepatic organ failures that is associated with increased mortality within a period of 28 days and up to 3 months from onset.[29–31] The organ failures that develop secondary to infection and lead to ACLF are discussed separately in the following sections.

Circulatory Failure and Shock

Patients with cirrhosis have hyperdynamic circulation, characterized by high cardiac output, relatively low arterial pressure, and low systemic vascular resistance. When infection develops in patients with cirrhosis, systemic circulation becomes even more hyperdynamic and hyporeactive to pharmacologic doses of alpha-adrenoreceptor agonists.[32,33] Patients with cirrhosis and septic shock have higher cardiac indices, higher plasma lactate concentrations, lower temperature, and higher mortality rates as compared with patients without cirrhosis.[34]

Renal Failure

Worsening systemic and splanchnic vasodilatation contributes to decreased effective circulating blood volume, which in turn activates the neuro hormonal mechanisms (rennin-angiotensin-aldosterone), triggering renal vasoconstriction and renal dysfunction. Up to 33% of patients with SBP develop renal failure and, similar to SBP, non-SBP infections precipitate renal failure in approximately one-third of patients with cirrhosis. The kidneys are the most common organs to fail in patients with cirrhosis with infection and worsening renal function is considered a key determinant of mortality in patients with cirrhosis.[30,35] Occurrence of Acute Kidney Injury (AKI) in patients with underlying liver disease and development of hepato-renal syndromes is discussed in more detail elsewhere in this issue (See Regner KR, Singbarti K: Kidney Injury in Liver Disease, in this issue).

Hepatic Encephalopathy

Infection is thought to be a major trigger of altered mental status and may result in cerebral edema.[36] Evidence that deterioration of neuropsychological test scores in patients with cirrhosis with SIRS that resolve with resolution of SIRS, suggest that SIRS mediators, such as NO and proinflammatory cytokines, may be important in modulating the cerebral effect of ammonia.[37] The development of hepatic encephalopathy in septic patients with cirrhosis is associated with worse prognosis.

Coagulopathy

Patients with liver disease have thrombocytopenia, platelet dysfunction, and decreased synthesis of coagulation factors. These coagulation abnormalities are more marked in patients with ongoing sepsis, likely secondary to worsening liver dysfunction. Further release of proinflammatory cytokines along with activation of the coagulation cascade leads to disseminated intravascular coagulation, a phenomenon commonly seen in patients with ACLF.[38]

Respiratory Failure

Pulmonary complications are common in patients with liver disease. Restricted expansion due to tense ascites and aspiration pneumonitis related to altered mental status further compromise an already vulnerable respiratory system.[39] At the cellular level there is reduced bactericidal activity of alveolar macrophages and alteration in lymphocyte subsets. In the presence of widespread immune dysfunction, these factors contribute to higher incidence of adult respiratory distress syndrome (ARDS) in cirrhosis.[40,41] Patients with cirrhosis and sepsis are more likely to die with ARDS compared to individuals with ARDS who did not have cirrhosis. Patients with cirrhosis requiring mechanical ventilation have mortality rates well above 50% and as high as 100% in one series.[42,43]

MANAGEMENT OF INFECTIONS IN LIVER DISEASE

Hospitalized patients with liver disease should be followed closely for development of any new signs or symptoms of infection. A complete diagnostic workup to rule out any infectious source should be completed in every patient with cirrhosis. If infection is suspected or confirmed, a prompt management strategy to counter hemodynamic and immune derangements should be instituted (**Fig. 2**).

General Approach to Management of Infections in Liver Disease

Universal management to any patient with underlying infection begins with prompt assessment of hemodynamic and respiratory status. Immediate control of the source of infection is paramount.

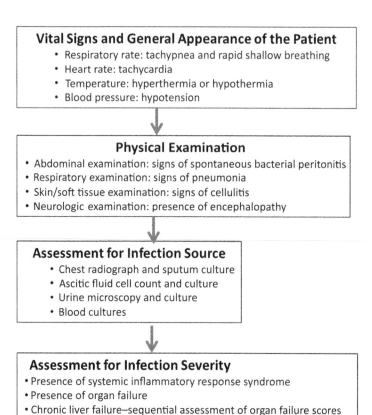

Vital Signs and General Appearance of the Patient
- Respiratory rate: tachypnea and rapid shallow breathing
- Heart rate: tachycardia
- Temperature: hyperthermia or hypothermia
- Blood pressure: hypotension

Physical Examination
- Abdominal examination: signs of spontaneous bacterial peritonitis
- Respiratory examination: signs of pneumonia
- Skin/soft tissue examination: signs of cellulitis
- Neurologic examination: presence of encephalopathy

Assessment for Infection Source
- Chest radiograph and sputum culture
- Ascitic fluid cell count and culture
- Urine microscopy and culture
- Blood cultures

Assessment for Infection Severity
- Presence of systemic inflammatory response syndrome
- Presence of organ failure
- Chronic liver failure–sequential assessment of organ failure scores

Fig. 2. Suggested workup in the diagnosis of bacterial infections in cirrhosis.

Hemodynamic resuscitation
There remains a lack of data on the best method of provision of resuscitation to patients with cirrhosis and severe infections. It is prudent to treat severe sepsis and septic shock in patients with cirrhosis following the same guidelines that are used for the general population. Goals of resuscitation should be achievement of euvolemia and adequate organ perfusion.[20] Vasopressor support should be initiated if significant hypotension persists despite adequate fluid resuscitation. Norepinephrine is the first line of vasopressor support in septic shock with vasopressin being the second-line therapy.[39,44]

Albumin
A decrease in mortality rates and reduced incidence of renal failure was observed with intravenous administration of 20% albumin in patients with cirrhosis and SBP.[45] Possible proposed mechanisms for improvement are due to albumin's oncotic properties, immunomodulatory and antioxidant effects, and its endothelium stabilization capacity.[46] After adjustment for other prognostic factors, albumin administration emerged as an independent predictor of survival in another study.[47] The use of intravenous albumin resuscitation may be associated with decreased mortality in patients with septic shock as compared with other resuscitation solutions[48]; however, there are no randomized control trials comparing albumin with other plasma expanders in patients with liver disease.

Hydrocortisone
Prevalence of relative adrenal insufficiency is high in patients with cirrhosis and septic shock, ranging from 51% to 77%.[49] In a recent study, low cortisol level was associated with impairments of circulatory and renal function, higher likelihood of development of severe sepsis and type I HRS, as well as higher short-term mortality.[50] Although the occurrence of relative adrenal insufficiency appears to be exaggerated in patients with cirrhosis and septic shock, whether replacement doses of hydrocortisone affect outcome remains unknown.

Nutritional support
Increased circulating TNF and leptin lead to anorexia, delayed gastric emptying, ascites, high bilirubin and cholestasis and high catabolic demands, and lead to nutritional compromise and poor outcomes.[51,52] A general approach to nutritional supplementation as in the general population with use of nutrition-dense formulas should be targeted, but it should be used carefully in patients with underlying ileus.

Approach to Antibiotic Therapy

It is imperative to administer antibiotics early when infections are suspected in patients with cirrhosis. Selection of empirical antibiotics treatment should ideally be based on infection type and severity as well as epidemiologic risk factors for development of resistant microorganisms. In general, it is prudent to start out with broad-spectrum antibiotics tailored to local epidemiology and then narrow as culture results return.

Third-generation cephalosporins continue to be the standard antibiotic treatment of many of the infections acquired in the community.[5,53] However, the empirical treatment of nosocomial and health care–associated (HCA) infections needs to be tailored with reference to the local epidemiologic pattern of multidrug-resistant bacteria.[54] Unsuitable choice of initial antibiotics, multidrug-resistant bacterial infections, and delayed start of appropriate antibiotics leads to failure of treatment and increased mortality. In one investigation, 7.2% of patients with cirrhosis and septic shock did not receive appropriate antibiotic therapy until death.[54–56]

Antibiotic Prophylaxis

Although essential in some cohorts with cirrhosis, antibiotic prophylaxis must be restricted to selected patients at high risk of developing bacterial infections. This is essential to prevent the development of antibiotic resistance.

Gastrointestinal bleeding
Patients with cirrhosis with upper gastrointestinal bleeding are predisposed to develop SBP and other infections during or immediately after the bleeding episode. The main risk period is the first 7 days after the hemorrhage, during which antibiotic prophylaxis is recommended. Oral norfloxacin is the first choice because of low cost and ease of administration.[20] Prophylaxis should be initiated as soon as possible, preferably before or immediately after completion of endoscopy. In addition, individual patient characteristics and local antibiotic susceptibility patterns should be considered before initiating antibiotic prophylaxis. Third-generation cephalosporins are recommended in patients with advanced cirrhosis, in those with a recent infection due to a quinolone-resistant organism, and those receiving quinolone prophylaxis.[57]

Primary prophylaxis (preventing first episode of spontaneous bacterial peritonitis)
The highest rates of first episode of SBP are observed in patients who, in addition to a low ascites total protein, have markers of severe liver failure (Child-Pugh score >9 points with serum bilirubin >3 mg/dL) and/or circulatory dysfunction

(serum creatinine >1.2 mg/dL, blood urea nitrogen >25 mg/dL, or serum sodium<130 mEq/L). One-year probability of developing SBP decreased from 61% to 7% in the group randomized to norfloxacin in a randomized trial of prophylaxis.[58] Long-term norfloxacin prophylaxis is therefore recommended with the previously mentioned risk factors with ciprofloxacin as an alternative in countries in which it is unavailable.[57]

Secondary prophylaxis (preventing recurrence of spontaneous bacterial peritonitis)

Patients who have recovered from a previous episode of SBP are at a very high risk of SBP recurrence in the absence of antibiotic prophylaxis. In this double-blind placebo-controlled randomized controlled trial, patients receiving norfloxacin had a 1-year probability of SBP recurrence of 20% versus 60% in patients treated with placebo.[59]

SPECIAL CONSIDERATIONS
Spontaneous Bacterial Peritonitis

SBP carries a poor prognosis, and hospital mortality ranges from 10% to 50%.[60,61] It is the most frequently seen bacterial infection in hospitalized patients with cirrhosis.[3] Survival relies on timely diagnosis and management of the infection. Increased predisposition of SBP in patients with cirrhosis is a result of intestinal overgrowth, bacterial translocation, altered intestinal mucosal barrier with increased permeability, and altered local immune response.[62] Diagnosis of SBP is dependent on ascitic fluid sampling. A polymorphonuclear cell count greater than 250 cells/mm^3 without evidence of an intra-abdominal surgically treatable source of infection is diagnostic.[63] The most common SBP isolates are *Escherichia coli, Klebsiella pneumoniae*, and *Streptococcus pneumoniae*.[63] Cefotaxime confers effective coverage against 95% of the ascitic/gut flora, including the 3 most common organisms. Alternatively, cephalosporins, such as ceftriaxone and ceftazidime, have been shown to be as effective.[64] Duration of therapy is at least 5 days with reported similar outcomes of 5 versus 10 days of antibiotic therapy.[65] Secondary prevention of SBP always should be considered in high-risk patients, as mentioned previously.

Importance of Fungal Infections

Fungal infections in patients with underlying liver disease are associated with very high mortality. Dysfunctional immune system, instrumentation, and corticosteroid therapy in sepsis and alcoholic hepatitis are the main risk factors for developing invasive fungal infections in this patient group. A recent retrospective study reported a mortality of 100% in patients with alcoholic hepatitis admitted to an intensive care unit if invasive mycoses developed. Invasive aspergillosis and candidemia were prominent infections. Mechanical ventilation, instrumentation, hemodialysis, and number of antibiotics used were some of the risk factors identified in the study.[66]

In another recent retrospective review of 185 patients by Alexopoulou and colleagues,[67] prevalence of fungal infections was 6% and 1-month mortality close to 90%. Fungal infections are difficult to diagnose in peritoneal fluid analysis, are usually fatal, and require a high index of suspicion. In addition, many first-line medications for these infections have hepatotoxic and nephrotoxic side effects, thus making appropriate treatment a challenge.

SUMMARY

Cirrhosis is a state of immune dysfunction with enhanced susceptibility to infection. Once infections occur, there is a high risk of death and/or the occurrence of complications, such as ACLF and other organ failures. The diagnosis of infections in cirrhosis is challenging and requires a high degree of clinical suspicion. Hospitalized patients with cirrhosis should be presumed to have an infection unless proven otherwise.

REFERENCES

1. Garcia-Tsao G. Bacterial infections in cirrhosis. Can J Gastroenterol 2004;18(6): 405–6.
2. Aggarwal A, Ong JP, Younossi ZM, et al. Predictors of mortality and resource utilization in cirrhotic patients admitted to the medical ICU. Chest 2001;119(5): 1489–97.
3. Fernandez J, Navasa M, Gomez J, et al. Bacterial infections in cirrhosis: epidemiological changes with invasive procedures and norfloxacin prophylaxis. Hepatology 2002;35:140–8.
4. Fernandez J, Acevedo J, Castro M, et al. Prevalence and risk factors of infections by multiresistant bacteria in cirrhosis: a prospective study. Hepatology 2012; 55(5):1551–61.
5. Merli M, Lucidi C, Giannelli V, et al. Cirrhotic patients are at risk for health care-associated bacterial infections. Clin Gastroenterol Hepatol 2010;8:979–85.
6. Borzio M, Salerno F, Piantoni L, et al. Bacterial infection in patients with advanced cirrhosis: a multicentre prospective study. Dig Liver Dis 2001;33:41–8.
7. D'Amico G, de Franchis R, Dell'Era A, editors. Variceal hemorrhage. New York: Springer Science+Business Media; 2014. p. 15.
8. Arvaniti V, D'Amico G, Fede G, et al. Infections in patients with cirrhosis increase mortality four-fold and should be used in determining prognosis. Gastroenterology 2010;139(4):1246–56.e1–e5.
9. Farhadi A, Gundlapalli S, Shaikh M, et al. Susceptibility to gut leakiness: a possible mechanism for endotoxaemia in non-alcoholic steatohepatitis. Liver Int 2008;28(7):1026–33.
10. Wade J, Rolando N, Philpott-Howard J, et al. Timing and aetiology of bacterial infections in a liver intensive care unit. J Hosp Infect 2003;53(2):144–6.
11. Antoniades CG, Berry PA, Davies ET, et al. Reduced monocyte HLA-DR expression: a novel biomarker of disease severity and outcome in acetaminophen-induced acute liver failure. Hepatology 2006;44(1):34–43.
12. Vaquero J, Polson J, Chung C, et al. Infection and the progression of hepatic encephalopathy in acute liver failure. Gastroenterology 2003;125(3):755–64.
13. Karvellas CJ, Pink F, McPhail M, et al. Predictors of bacteraemia and mortality in patients with acute liver failure. Intensive Care Med 2009;35(8):1390–6.
14. Leber B, Spindelboeck W, Stadlbauer V, et al. Infectious complications of acute and chronic liver disease. Semin Respir Crit Care Med 2012;33(1):80–95.
15. Sun HY, Cacciarelli TV, Singh N. Impact of pretransplant infections on clinical outcomes of liver transplant recipients. Liver Transpl 2010;16(2):222–8.
16. Weiss E, Dahmani S, Bert F, et al. Early-onset pneumonia after liver transplantation: microbiological findings and therapeutic consequences. Liver Transpl 2010; 16(10):1178–85.
17. Jalan R, Fernandez J, Wiest R, et al. Bacterial infections in cirrhosis: a position statement based on the EASL Special Conference 2013. J Hepatol 2014;60(6): 1310–24.
18. Bajaj JS, O'Leary JG, Reddy KR, et al. Second infections independently increase mortality in hospitalized patients with cirrhosis: the North American consortium for

the study of end-stage liver disease (NACSELD) experience. Hepatology 2012; 56:2328–35.

19. Albillos A, Lario M, Alvarez-Mon M. Cirrhosis-associated immune dysfunction: distinctive features and clinical relevance. J Hepatol 2014;61:1385–96.

20. Fernandez J, Gustot T. Management of bacterial infections in cirrhosis. J Hepatol 2012;56:S1–12.

21. Gabay C, Kushner I. Acute-phase proteins and other systemic responses to inflammation. N Engl J Med 1999;340:448–54.

22. Cervoni JP, Thévenot T, Weil D, et al. C-reactive protein predicts short-term mortality in patients with cirrhosis. J Hepatol 2012;56:1299–304.

23. Tsiakalos A, Karatzaferis A, Ziakas P, et al. Acute-phase proteins as indicators of bacterial infection in patients with cirrhosis. Liver Int 2009;29:1538–42.

24. Papp M, Vitalis Z, Altorjay I, et al. Acute phase proteins in the diagnosis and prediction of cirrhosis associated bacterial infections. Liver Int 2012;32:603–11.

25. Wacker C, Prkno A, Brunkhorst FM, et al. Procalcitonin as a diagnostic marker for sepsis: a systematic review and meta-analysis. Lancet Infect Dis 2013;13: 426–35.

26. Schuetz P, Albrich W, Mueller B. Procalcitonin for diagnosis of infection and guide to antibiotic decisions: past, present and future. BMC Med 2011;22:107.

27. Cholongitas E, Papatheodoridis GV, Lahanas A, et al. Increasing frequency of gram-positive bacteria in spontaneous bacterial peritonitis. Liver Int 2005;25(1): 57–61.

28. Viasus D, Garcia-Vidal C, Castellote J, et al. Community-acquired pneumonia in patients with liver cirrhosis: clinical features, outcomes, and usefulness of severity scores. Medicine (Baltimore) 2011;90(2):110–8.

29. Moreau R, Jalan R, Gines P, et al. Acute-on chronic liver failure is a distinct syndrome that develops in patients with acute decompensation of cirrhosis. Gastroenterology 2013;144:1426–37.

30. Jalan R, Yurdaydin C, Bajaj JS, et al, World Gastroenterology Organization Working Party. Toward an improved definition of acute-on-chronic liver failure. Gastroenterology 2014;147:4–10.

31. Bajaj JS, O'Leary JG, Reddy KR, et al, North American Consortium For The Study Of End-Stage Liver Disease (NACSELD). Survival in infection-related acute-on-chronic liver failure is defined by extrahepatic organ failures. Hepatology 2014; 60:250–6.

32. Moreau R, Lee SS, Soupison T, et al. Abnormal tissue oxygenation in patients with cirrhosis and liver failure. J Hepatol 1988;7:98–105.

33. Ruiz-del-Arbol L, Urman J, Fernandez J, et al. Systemic, renal, and hepatic hemodynamic derangement in cirrhotic patients with spontaneous bacterial peritonitis. Hepatology 2003;38:1210–8.

34. Moreau R, Hadengue A, Soupison T, et al. Septic shock in patients with cirrhosis: hemodynamic and metabolic characteristics and intensive care unit outcome. Crit Care Med 1992;20:746–50.

35. Terra C, Guevara M, Torre A, et al. Renal failure in patients with cirrhosis and sepsis unrelated to spontaneous bacterial peritonitis: value of MELD score. Gastroenterology 2005;129:1944–53.

36. Merli M, Lucidi C, Pentassuglio I, et al. Increased risk of cognitive impairment in cirrhotic patients with bacterial infections. J Hepatol 2013;59(2):243–50.

37. Shawcross DL, Davies NA, Williams R, et al. Systemic inflammatory response exacerbates the neuropsychological effects of induced hyperammonemia in cirrhosis. J Hepatol 2004;40:247–54.

38. Plessier A, Denninger MH, Consigny Y, et al. Coagulation disorders in patients with cirrhosis and severe sepsis. Liver Int 2003;23:440–8.

39. Gustot T, Durand F, Lebrec D, et al. Severe sepsis in cirrhosis. Hepatology 2009; 50(6):2022–33.

40. Wallaert B, Aerts C, Colombel JF, et al. Human alveolar macrophage antibacterial activity in the alcoholic lung. Am Rev Respir Dis 1991;144:278–83.

41. Wallaert B, Colombel JF, Prin L, et al. Bronchoalveolar lavage in alcoholic liver cirrhosis. T-lymphocyte subsets and immunoglobulin concentrations. Chest 1992;101:468–73.

42. Monchi M, Bellenfant F, Cariou A, et al. Early predictive factors of survival in the acute respiratory distress syndrome. A multivariate analysis. Am J Respir Crit Care Med 1998;158:1076–81.

43. Rabe C, Schmitz V, Paashaus M, et al. Does intubation really equal death in cirrhotic patients? Factors influencing outcome in patients with liver cirrhosis requiring mechanical ventilation. Intensive Care Med 2004;30:1564–71.

44. De Backer D, Biston P, Devriendt J, et al. SOAP II Investigators. Comparison of dopamine and norepinephrine in the treatment of shock. N Engl J Med 2010; 362:779–89.

45. Sort P, Navasa M, Arroyo V, et al. Effect of intravenous albumin on renal impairment and mortality in patients with cirrhosis and spontaneous bacterial peritonitis. N Engl J Med 1999;341:403–9.

46. Garcia-Martinez R, Caraceni P, Bernardi M, et al. Albumin: pathophysiologic basis of its role in the treatment of cirrhosis and its complications. Hepatology 2013;58(5):1836–46.

47. Guevara M, Terra C, Nazar A, et al. Albumin for bacterial infections other than spontaneous bacterial peritonitis in cirrhosis. A randomized, controlled study. J Hepatol 2012;57:759–65.

48. Delaney AP, Dan A, McCaffrey J, et al. The role of albumin as a resuscitation fluid for patients with sepsis: a systematic review and metaanalysis. Crit Care Med 2011;39:386–91.

49. Fede G, Spadaro L, Tomaselli T, et al. Adrenocortical dysfunction in liver disease: a systematic review. Hepatology 2012;55:1282–91.

50. Acevedo J, Fernández J, Prado V, et al. Relative adrenal insufficiency in decompensated cirrhosis: relationship to short-term risk of severe sepsis, hepatorenal syndrome, and death. Hepatology 2013;58:1757–65.

51. Krenitsky J. Nutrition for patients with hepatic failure. Pract Gastroenterol 2003;6: 23–42.

52. Tsien CD, McCullough AJ, Dasarathy S. Late evening snack: exploiting a period of anabolic opportunity in cirrhosis. J Gastroenterol Hepatol 2012;27:430–41.

53. Song JY, Jung SJ, Park CW, et al. Prognostic significance of infection acquisition sites in spontaneous bacterial peritonitis: nosocomial vs. community acquired. J Korean Med Sci 2006;21:666–71.

54. Fernandez J, Arroyo V. Bacterial infections in cirrhosis–a growing problem with significant implications. Clin Liver Dis 2013;2:102–5.

55. Ginès P, Angeli P, Lenz K, et al. EASL clinical practice guidelines on the management of ascites, spontaneous bacterial peritonitis, and hepatorenal syndrome in cirrhosis. J Hepatol 2010;53:397–417.

56. Arabi YM, Dara SI, Memish Z, et al. Antimicrobial therapeutic determinants of outcomes from septic shock among patients with cirrhosis. Hepatology 2012; 56(6):2305–15.

57. de Franchis R, Baveno VI Faculty. Expanding consensus in portal hypertension. Report of the Baveno VI Consensus Workshop: stratifying risk and individualizing care for portal hypertension. J Hepatol 2015;63:743–52.

58. Fernandez J, Navasa N, Planas R, et al. Primary prophylaxis of spontaneous bacterial peritonitis delays hepatorenal syndrome and improves survival in cirrhosis. Gastroenterology 2007;133:818–24.

59. Gines P, Rimola A, Planas R, et al. Norfloxacin prevents spontaneous bacterial peritonitis recurrence in cirrhosis: results of a double-blind, placebo-controlled trial. Hepatology 1990;12:716–24.

60. Pinzello G, Simonetti RG, Craxi A, et al. Spontaneous bacterial peritonitis: a prospective investigation in predominantly nonalcoholic cirrhotic patients. Hepatology 1983;3:545e9.

61. Nobre SR, Cabral JE, Gomes JJ, et al. In-hospital mortality in spontaneous bacterial peritonitis: a new predictive model. Eur J Gastroenterol Hepatol 2008; 20:1176e81.

62. Berg RD. Bacterial translocation from the gastrointestinal tract. Adv Exp Med Biol 1999;473:11–30.

63. Runyon BA, Practice Guidelines Committee, American Association for the Study of Liver Diseases (AASLD). Management of adult patients with ascites due to cirrhosis. Hepatology 2004;39:841–56.

64. Rimola A, García-Tsao G, Navasa M, et al. Diagnosis, treatment and prophylaxis of spontaneous bacterial peritonitis: a consensus document. International Ascites Club. J Hepatol 2000;32:142–53.

65. Arroyo V, Bataller R, Ginès P. Spontaneous bacterial peritonitis. In: O'Grady JG, Lake JR, editors. Comprehensive clinical hepatology. 1st edition. Barcelona (Spain): Mosby; 2000. p. 7.10–4.

66. Lahmer T, Messer M, Schwerdtfeger C, et al. Invasive mycosis in medical intensive care unit patients with severe alcoholic hepatitis. Mycopathologia 2014; 177(3–4):193–7.

67. Alexopoulou A, Vasilieva L, Agiasotelli D, et al. Fungal infections in patients with cirrhosis. J Hepatol 2015;63(4):1043–5.

The Liver in Critical Illness

Tessa W. Damm, DO[a],*, David J. Kramer, MD[b,c]

KEYWORDS

- Acute liver failure (ALF) • Acute-on-chronic liver failure (ACLF) • Critical illness
- Multiple organ failure (MOF) • Intracranial hypertension (IH)
- Acute respiratory distress syndrome (ARDS)

KEY POINTS

- Kupffer cell dysfunction as a result of chronic liver disease or in the setting of acute hepatic insult results in inadequate endotoxin clearance and is a driver of multiple organ failure (MOF).
- Hepatic encephalopathy that progresses to cerebral edema with intracranial hypertension in acute liver failure warrants intracranial pressure monitoring in select patients.
- Treatment of acutely increased intracranial pressure includes administration of hypertonic saline or mannitol.
- Volume resuscitation is often warranted in the vasodilated hyperdynamic state that characterizes liver failure; an intervention that requires ongoing monitoring of objective endpoints including central venous pressure, stroke volume variation, and bedside echocardiography.

INTRODUCTION

The liver has long been known to play a central role in critical illness. Hippocrates appreciated that jaundice portends a poor prognosis and that this process can result from either direct hepatic injury or nonhepatic systemic illness **Boxes 1** and **2**.[1] Centuries later the role of the liver as a significant contributor in host defenses was further elucidated, this time with the additional hypothesis that liver dysfunction is a driver of multiple organ failure (MOF).[1,2] This article reviews pertinent anatomic and physiologic considerations of the liver in critical illness, followed by a selective review of associated organ dysfunction.

CAUSES OF LIVER DISEASE

Depending on the specific cause of acute liver failure (ALF), its presentation may vary from one without precedent signs or symptoms to one with an associated prodromal

[a] Critical Care Medicine & Neurocritical Care, Aurora Critical Care Service, Milwaukee, WI, USA; [b] Aurora Critical Care Service, Milwaukee, WI, USA; [c] University of Wisconsin, School of Medicine and Public Health, Madison, WI, USA
* Corresponding author. 2901 West Kinnickinnic River Parkway, Suite 315, Milwaukee, WI 53215.
E-mail address: tessa.damm@aurora.org

Crit Care Clin 32 (2016) 425–438
http://dx.doi.org/10.1016/j.ccc.2016.02.002
0749-0704/16/$ – see front matter © 2016 Elsevier Inc. All rights reserved.

Box 1
Modified KCH Criteria (acetaminophen or paracetamol [APAP] intoxication)

Strongly consider listing for transplant if: Arterial lactate level greater than 3.5 mmol/L after early fluid resuscitation

List for transplant if: Arterial pH less than 7.3 or lactate level greater than 3.0 mmol/L after adequate fluid resuscitation

List for transplant if all 3 occur within 24-hour period: Serum creatinine level greater than 300 mol/L; INR greater than 6.5 (prothrombin time >100 seconds); Grade III/IV encephalopathy

From Bernal W, Donaldson N, Wyncoll D, et al. Blood lactate as an early predictor of outcome in paracetamol-induced acute liver failure: a cohort study. Lancet 2002;359(9306):562; with permission.

---

illness. Regardless of cause, liver failure and resultant hepatocyte dysfunction are directly linked to impaired host immune function, protein synthesis, and clearance of activated clotting factors.[3]

Kupffer cells (KC), or macrophages resident in liver sinusoids, comprise 80% to 90% of all tissue macrophages within the body and serve as the main site of clearance of particles from the bloodstream.[3,4] Anatomically, KC are positioned to serve as the first line of defense against bacteria, endotoxins, and microbial debris from the gastrointestinal (GI) tract, which are then delivered to the liver via the portal vein. The splanchnic circulation receives 25% of cardiac output; blood volume that subsequently circulates through an extensive network of hepatic sinusoidal microvasculature. The resultant blood-cell contact time results in consistent and effective hepatic clearance.[2]

In the setting of liver dysfunction, impaired KC endotoxin clearance results in increased blood-level presentation of microbial debris to other cells within the reticuloendothelial system, including splenic, pulmonary alveolar, and bony macrophages; a sequence referred to as spillover.[3] These extrahepatic reticuloendothelial sites are ill equipped to handle the full burden of endotoxin clearance. The result is a complex and interrelated sequence of inadequate endotoxin clearance and subsequent organ dysfunction, and this is summarized in **Fig. 1**.

Even in the setting of a previously healthy liver, the milieu of critical illness presents stress to previously functional hepatocytes as it exposes them to a mismatch between metabolic demand and hepatic blood flow. Critical illness, particularly illness that

---

Box 2
KCH criteria (non-APAP intoxication)

INR greater than 6.5 (PT >100)

Or at least of 3 of the following:

Age less than 11 years or greater than 40 years

Total bilirubin level greater than 17.6 mg/dL (300 μmol/L)

Interval between onset of jaundice and development of hepatic encephalopathy (HE) greater than 7 days

INR greater than 3.5 (PT >50)

Drug toxicity (non-APAP)

From O'Grady JG, Alexander GJ, Hayllar KM, et al. Early indicators of prognosis in fulminant hepatic failure. Gastroenterology 1989;97(2):443; with permission.

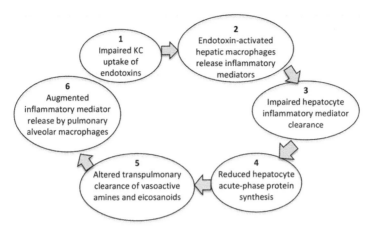

Fig. 1. The role of liver dysfunction in development of MOF. (*Data from* Matuschak GM, Rinaldo JE. Organ interactions in the adult respiratory distress syndrome during sepsis. Role of the liver in host defense. Chest 1988;94(2):400–6.)

results from sepsis, is thought to disrupt normal hepatic function. The mechanisms are related to altered blood flow to and within the liver, as seen in experimental models.[5–7] The alteration in sinusoidal blood flow coincides with an intense increase in metabolic demand by both hepatocytes and KC. Therapeutic interventions, including positive end-expiratory pressure (PEEP), or concurrent right ventricular dysfunction and tricuspid valvular regurgitation also serve to increase sinusoidal pressure.

Portal hypertension results from increased flow through a high-resistance network. In cirrhosis it is thought that this resistance is fixed and relates to scarring with distortion of the vasculature. It is probable that sinusoidal injury influences a dynamic and potentially modifiable component of resistance.[8]

Resultant splanchnic ischemia and impaired hepatic metabolism is difficult to measure early in its course by traditional liver function tests that assess solely for the presence or absence of hepatobiliary injury.[9] Gastric mucosal oxygenation can be indirectly measured by tonometry, which quantifies gastric intramucosal pH,[10,11] and a flow-dependent assessment of liver function exists in the monoethylglycinexy-lidide formation test.[12] Both tests provide earlier indications of impaired hepatocyte clearance and correlate with patient mortality,[10,13] although they are infrequently used in clinical practice.

SEVERITY OF LIVER DYSFUNCTION

Cirrhosis significantly increases all-cause mortality during hospitalization. Hospitalized patients with cirrhosis are more prone to sepsis and respiratory failure and are 3 times more likely to die in the hospital than noncirrhotic patients.[14] Mortality among patients with underlying cirrhosis and acutely decompensated acute disease requiring organ support in an intensive care unit (ICU) ranges from 50% to nearly 100%.[15] Accordingly, ICU-specific scoring systems have been evaluated for their accuracy in this patient population. The Acute Physiology and Chronic Health Evaluation II (APACHE II), Simplified Acute Physiology Score (SAPS II), and Simplified Organ Failure Assessment (SOFA) have been shown to be superior at predicting outcome compared with the liver-specific Child-Pugh score.[15] Universally, the presence of 3 or more organ failures in patients with cirrhosis correlated with ICU mortality of greater than 90%.[15]

The Model for End-Stage Liver Disease (MELD) score was originally designed to estimate survival in patients undergoing transjugular intrahepatic portosystemic shunting (TIPS).[16] In 2002 its use expanded and it remains the basis of prioritization for liver transplant and allocation in the United States. MELD takes into account serum creatinine level, total serum bilirubin level, and International Normalized Ratio (INR). This model has been validated to accurately predict short-term mortality (3 months) in patients waiting for liver transplant.[17]

MELD formula: $3.8 \times \log_e$ (bilirubin [mg/dL]) $+ 11.2 \times \log_e$ (INR) $+ 9.6 \times \log_e$ (creatinine [mg/dL])

Worldwide, the modified Kings College Hospital (KCH) criteria for ALF are used to list patients for liver transplant. MELD has been compared with KCH and has been shown to correlate equally for mortality.[16] A MELD of 32 is a sensitive (79%) and specific (71%) predictor of mortality in the same patient cohort.[16]

SELECTIVE REVIEW OF ORGAN DYSFUNCTION AND INTERVENTION
Neurologic

One of the most serious complications of ALF is HE that progresses to cerebral edema and intracranial hypertension (IH). Ammonia has been implicated as the driving pathophysiologic substance in the process because both serum and brain concentrations of ammonia and its primary metabolic product, glutamine, are found in high concentrations in encephalopathic patients.[18] A previous article discussed in detail the pathophysiology of enhanced blood-brain permeability, altered astrocyte function, and resultant cytotoxic edema. It is probable that the combination of systemic inflammatory response and hyperammonemia predisposes to cerebral edema and intracranial hypertension.[19]

In addition to increased brain edema, cerebral perfusion pressure (CPP) is often compromised in critical illness by the presence of arterial hypotension. Decreased mean arterial pressure (MAP) and increased intracranial pressure (ICP) both contribute to compromised CPP by the principle of the equation, CPP = MAP – ICP. Left unchecked, arterial hypotension and increased ICP can progress to result in ischemic brain damage and herniation.

Further perpetuating the issue of cerebral edema in ALF is the fact that cerebral vascular resistance (CVR) is decreased early in ALF by release of cerebral vasodilatory substances, which results in increased cerebral blood flow (CBF) in the following manner: CBF = CPP/CVR. The net result of increased CBF is increased brain delivery of circulating ammonia and cytokines.[20] The loss of autoregulation of CBF that is universal in ALF has been attributed to decreased functional hepatic mass.[21]

The presence of IH grossly correlates with degree of coma. However, physical examination maneuvers, including inspection of the pupils and fundi, may not reveal signs of edema until ICP is increased to 30 mm Hg. It is desirable to maintain ICP less than or equal to 20 to 25 mm Hg at all times, therefore proposed indications for invasive ICP in patients with ALF are well established (**Box 3**).

Invasive monitoring is associated with complications.[22] Patients at highest risk of IH are characterized by the combination of young age, hyperammonemia, and multiple-systems organ failure (renal failure requiring renal replacement therapy and

---

Box 3
Indications for ICP monitoring in patients with ALF

1. Patients who fulfill KCH criteria

2. Presence of pupillary abnormalities or seizures

3. Patients who fulfill 3 to 4 systemic inflammatory response syndrome criteria

4. Arterial ammonia concentration greater than 150 mmol/L

5. Low serum sodium concentration

6. Hemodynamic compromise requiring vasopressor support

7. Surrogate markers of extremes of cerebral blood flow (jugular oxygen saturations or transcranial Doppler monitoring)

Adapted from Larsen FS, Wendon J. Prevention and management of brain edema in patients with acute liver failure. Liver Transpl 2008;14 Suppl 2:S92; with permission.

---

hypotension requiring management with vasopressors).[23] For patients without high-risk features, invasive monitoring may not be outweighed by the risks of doing so. Ideally ICP monitoring is supplemented by monitoring of brain tissue oxygen saturation, because this more adequately assesses global and regional cerebral oxygenation in the setting of impaired CBF autoregulation.[24,25] Such monitoring can be accomplished by placement of a Licox catheter or bedside cerebral microdialysis, which analyses lactate/pyruvate ratios in the brain cortex.

Regardless of the type of monitoring device used, primary interventions to control IH include manipulation of body position, fluid therapy, vasopressor support, oxygenation and ventilation, and control of body temperature. Patients' bed heads should be maintained at greater than or equal to 30° of elevation with forward-facing head positions because avoidance of neck rotation and side bending enables optimal intracranial venous drainage.

Normovolemia should be attained by intravascular volume resuscitation with isotonic intravenous fluids as necessary. Volume expansion often results in increased arterial pressure and reversal of lactic acidosis. It is imperative to use objective end points of resuscitation, including central venous pressure (CVP) trends, stroke volume variation (SVV), and bedside echocardiography so as to avoid volume overload that may further perpetuate cerebral edema. Goal CPP is 60 to 80 mg Hg in ALF. If arterial hypotension persists despite appropriate volume resuscitation, vasoactive medications may be initiated. Choice of vasopressor is discussed later.

A low threshold should be maintained for intubation (Glasgow Coma Scale ≤8 or grade III/VI encephalopathy) to ensure appropriate oxygenation and ventilation. Hyperventilation is known to cause precapillary vasoconstriction that decreases CBF and ICP.[24] Although this may be intentionally instituted as a rescue maneuver for acute increases in ICP with signs of imminent herniation, it is not recommendation for routine application. Normocapnia ($Paco_2$ 35–40 mm Hg) is optimal for control of ICP, which must be balanced with desires for low-tidal-volume ventilation in patients with concurrent pulmonary complications. Arterial oxygen saturation should be maintained at greater than or equal to 95% because hypoxemia worsens outcomes.

Maintenance of normothermia is imperative in the setting of IH because fever increases CBF and oxidative metabolism. Therapeutic hypothermia (32°C–34°C) has been shown in experimental models to ameliorate brain edema and slow both systemic production and cerebral uptake of ammonia.[26] Potential consequences of prolonged hypothermia, including increased infectious complications, have limited its application to settings of refractory ICP requiring a short-term bridge to transplant.

Restoration of the osmotic pressure gradient through administration of hypertonic saline or mannitol remains the treatment of choice for reduction of increased ICP. Hypertonic saline may be preferred in patients with ALF because of its higher reflection coefficient and proof of ICP control in patients with ALF.[27] In addition, hypertonic saline is not associated with the osmotic diuresis that accompanies mannitol administration, which may serve to exacerbate intravascular volume depletion. Corticosteroids should not be used to treat the cytotoxic edema that characterizes IH.[28] Continuous renal replacement therapy, plasmapheresis, and extracorporeal albumin dialysis techniques remain experimental in their use to modulate the osmotic pressure gradient in ALF.

In addition, analgesia and sedation are often required to control ICP as well as to allow safe implementation of invasive ICP monitoring and mechanical ventilation. The gamma-aminobutyric acid hypothesis in the pathogenesis of HE is a reminder that increased drug binding sites enhance sensitivity to benzodiazepines and barbiturates in patients with ALF.[29] Continuous sedation is typically only required in extreme cases, including refractory IH or seizure. In such instances propofol has gained popularity for use because of its rapid onset, short duration of action, and antiepileptogenic properties. Hourly doses should not exceed 5 mg/kg of body weight so as to avoid risk of propofol infusion syndrome. More commonly, sedation may be administered as needed, with dose titration and frequency of administration based on the Richmond Agitation and Sedation Score. Selective use of analgesic agents with inactive metabolites such as fentanyl and hydromorphone is encouraged. Similarly, pain score–directed titration of bolus administration rather than continuous infusion is recommended in patients with HE to avoid worsening encephalopathy and impaired mobility leading to sarcopenia and debilitation.

Cardiovascular

Liver failure is most frequently associated with a vasodilated hyperdynamic state.[30,31] Volume resuscitation is often necessary as an initial measure in the management of arterial hypotension with reduced afterload. Objective end points of resuscitation, including CVP, SVV, and bedside echocardiography, are recommended. Serum chloride levels should drive selection of resuscitative fluid because, if patients are hyperchloremic, chloride-rich formulations (0.9% NaCl and 5% albumin) should be avoided due to the association of hyperchloremic metabolic acidosis with renal dysfunction and mortality.[32,33]

If arterial hypotension persists despite adequate volume expansion, norepinephrine is the vasopressor of choice to achieve sustained MAP greater than or equal to 65 mm Hg. All vasopressors must be initiated with the knowledge that the effect on CBF and ICP directly follows changes in arterial pressure because of loss of cerebral autoregulation.[24] Unlike other vasoactive agents, terlipressin has been shown to increase CPP and CBF but not to alter ICP[34] and therefore should be considered a valuable additive agent where available for use. If terlipressin is not available, vasopressin is an acceptable additive agent to hypotension unresponsive to norepinephrine.[28] An initial management approach to patients with liver disease admitted to the ICU is detailed in **Fig. 2**.

Additional points germane to care of critically ill patients with liver dysfunction are as follows:

- Central venous saturation (SCVo$_2$) is a less reliable marker of resuscitation because oxygen consumption is lower in acute and chronic liver dysfunction, making SCVo$_2$ high at baseline.[35]

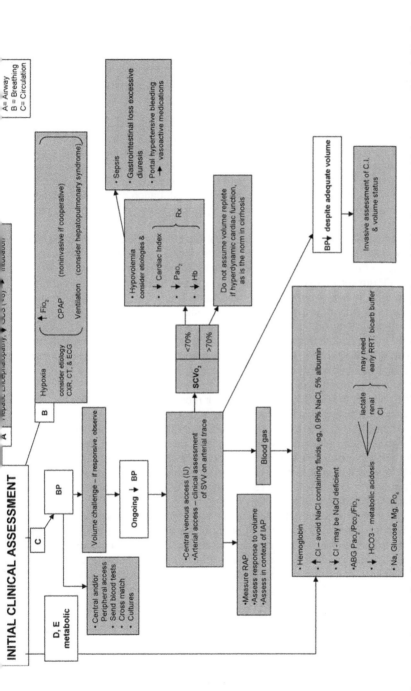

Fig. 2. Management approaches for patients with cirrhosis who are admitted to the ICU. ABG, arterial blood gases; BP, blood pressure; bicarb, bicarbonate; C.I., cardiac index; CPAP, continuous positive airway pressure; CT, computed tomography; CXR, chest radiograph; ECG, echocardiogram; Fio$_2$, fraction of inspired oxygen; GCS, Glasgow Coma Scale; Hb, hemoglobin; HPS, hepatopulmonary syndrome; IAP, intra-abdominal pressure; IJ, internal jugular; PA, pulmonary artery; PCWP, pulmonary capillary wedge pressure; PPH, portopulmonary hypertension; RAP, right atrial pressure; RRT, renal replacement therapy; Rx, treat; SCVo$_2$, central venous oxygen saturation. (*From* Olson JC, Wendon J, Kramer DJ, et al. Intensive care of the patient with cirrhosis. Hepatology 2011;54(5):1868; with permission.)

- Hepatic dysfunction and endotoxemia are both associated with delayed lactate clearance.[36] This alteration is independent of liver hypoperfusion and mitigates the routine use of lactate clearance as an end point of resuscitation in this patient population.
- Acid-base disturbances are common in critical illness with ALF. The anion gap corrected for albumin, phosphate, and lactate correlates well with strong ion difference, although this has not been associated with hospital mortality.[37]

Respiratory

A previous article addressed in detail respiratory complications of cirrhosis including hepatopulmonary syndrome and portopulmonary hypertension. Critically ill patients with liver disease are also at increased risk for pneumonia, pleural effusions, atelectasis, cardiogenic pulmonary edema, and acute respiratory distress syndrome (ARDS). It is worth restating that a low threshold for intubation should be maintained in ALF with HE because both hypoxemia and hypercapnia are associated with worse outcomes.

Ideally mechanical ventilation should be governed by principles unique to the milieu of liver failure. Permissive hypercapnia should be carefully avoided in patients with IH as vasodilatory effects of $PaCO_2$ on cerebral vasculature result in increased ICP. High doses of PEEP are known to decrease venous return with modest resultant decreases in cardiac output. In experimental models the same amount of PEEP has been shown to have more significant hemodynamic manifestations on splanchnic hypoperfusion, with measurable decreases in hepatic, portal, and mesenteric blood flow.[38] Application of PEEP in this patient population therefore should aim to minimize hemodynamic insults to splanchnic perfusion while also offsetting the right ventricular dysfunction that often develops in the setting of portopulmonary hypertension.

The compromised systemic and pulmonary defenses that characterize ALF both predispose patients to ARDS and modulate their recovery from the syndrome.[39] Supportive care including low-tidal-volume mechanical ventilation targeting plateau pressures less than 30 cm H_2O is recommended. Increased intra-abdominal pressure secondary to ascites may need to be addressed via large-volume paracentesis to improve pulmonary compliance. ARDS secondary to end-stage liver failure (ESLF) is irreversible and universally fatal.[39] However, a small series focused on carefully selected patients in whom ARDS was secondary to ESLF showed successful reversal of ARDS after orthotopic liver transplant.[40]

Hepatic hydrothorax commonly develops in the setting of acute illness. This condition may be managed medically by control of ascites through sodium restriction and diuresis as hemodynamics allow. Thoracentesis may be necessary, but chest tube placement should be avoided because persistent drainage places patients at risk for hypovolemia, hemorrhage, and infection. As in non–acutely ill patients, hydrothorax refractory to medical management is an indication for TIPS. However, the increased risk of subsequent encephalopathy following TIPS often limits the utility of this intervention in the setting of acute illness.

Renal

Renal failure complicating ALF portends a poor prognosis. As such, tenets of critical care in ALF include avoidance of nephrotoxic medications and circumstances resulting in decreased renal perfusion. Intravascular volume depletion should be avoided. Tense ascites should be relieved before it precipitates abdominal compartment syndrome. Monitor for increased abdominal pressure and perform large-volume paracentesis with concurrent albumin replacement (6–8 g albumin per liter of ascites removed) as indicated to maintain bladder pressure less than 20 mm Hg.[41]

Specific therapy for hepatorenal syndrome, as discussed in a prior article, includes volume expansion and vasoconstrictor therapy as well as prompt consideration for simultaneous liver-kidney transplant. Renal replacement therapy may be indicated as a bridge to transplant in treating volume overload, electrolyte disturbances, and refractory acidosis. Novel uses of renal replacement therapy in ALF include reduction of circulating level of ammonia and thermoregulation.[42]

Hepatic

ALF or acute-on-chronic liver failure (ACLF) should prompt investigation of superimposed injury, including new viral infection, APAP or other toxicity, alcoholic hepatitis, or portal vein thrombosis. Acute decompensation may also be secondary to extrahepatic insult, including infection, variceal bleeding, or trauma. The PIRO (predisposition, injury, response, organ) concept has been proposed as a systematic manner in which to evaluate such patients, and is summarized in **Fig. 3**.[43]

Targeted therapies for specific diagnoses include glucocorticoids or pentoxifylline in alcoholic hepatitis, although neither was associated with mortality benefit in a recent study.[44] N-acetylcysteine (NAC) remains the standard of care for APAP-induced ALF. NAC has also been used in non–APAP-induced ALF with proven mortality benefit.[45] Current practice dictates administration of NAC in all cases of drug-related hepatotoxicity, suspect mushroom poisoning, and idiopathic ALF.[28]

Gastrointestinal/Nutrition

ALF is a catabolic state and protein calorie malnutrition is common. Early and consistent enteral nutrition is paramount, although the optimal formulation has not been established. Theoretic concerns regarding high protein loads causing worsening

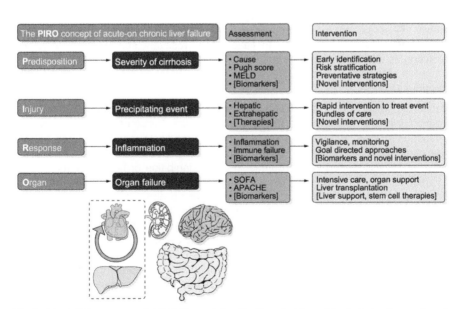

Fig. 3. The PIRO concept of ACLF. (*From* Jalan R, Gines P, Olson JC, et al. Acute-on chronic liver failure. J Hepatol 2012;57(6):1340; with permission.)

hyperammonemia have not been substantiated. The current recommendation is to prioritize early enteral feeding with a normal quantity of protein (0.8–1.2 g/kg/d).

In advanced liver disease, impaired gluconeogenesis and glycogen storage make patients prone to hypoglycemia. This possibility should be regularly monitored and treated with dextrose infusion when present. Vitamin supplementation with intravenous thiamine (100 mg intravenously daily for 3 to 5 days) and trace elements, primarily zinc (25–50 mg 3 times a day), has also been recommended.[41]

All patients with ALF in the ICU should receive stress ulcer prophylaxis with histamine blocking agents or proton pump inhibitors because they are at increased risk for GI bleed.[28] If upper GI bleeding does occur, in addition to supportive care and reversal of coagulopathy, including vitamin K supplementation, patients should be treated with empiric antibiotics because these have been associated with reduction in bacterial infections, all-cause mortality, rebleeding events, and hospital length of stay.[46]

Coagulation

Correction of coagulation abnormalities in the absence of bleeding or before ICU procedures is not indicated. Functional assays, including thromboelastography (TEG) and thromboelastometry (ROTEM) provide information regarding clot development reflective of in vivo hemostasis and should be used to guide product replacement when necessary. TEG also readily assesses fibrinolysis, which, if present outside of disseminated intravascular coagulation, should be treated with aminocaproic acid or tranexamic acid. Active bleeding in the setting of thrombocytopenia warrants platelet transfusion to maintain a level greater than 50×10^9/L. Qualitative platelet dysfunction may be attenuated by the administration of desmopressin (desamino-D-arginine vasopressin).

Endocrine

Among patients with cirrhosis and severe sepsis, more than 50% have adrenal insufficiency.[47] Assessment for cortisol deficiency and treatment with stress-dose hydrocortisone (50 mg every 6 hours) in vasopressor-resistant shock improves shock resolution as well as patient survival.[48]

Infectious Disease

Infectious complications of ALF are common and often multifactorial secondary to impaired immune function, increased propensity for translocation of gut flora in advanced cirrhosis, and high necessity of invasive medical procedures in this patient population. Development of infection is also of significant prognostic importance because it is associated with progression of HE, inhibition of hepatic regeneration, reduction of rates of successful transplant, and increased morbidity and mortality.[42] Minimal evaluation includes blood cultures; urinalysis and culture if indicated; and aspiration of ascites for culture, cell count, and differential as well as albumin, total protein, and cytology. Patients with a large serum-ascites albumin gap are at increased risk of subsequent spontaneous bacterial peritonitis.

Common practice is to maintain a very low threshold for initiation of empiric antibiotics as well as antifungal therapy at the time of admission in patients with HE or any other evidence of organ dysfunction. Duration of therapy is subsequently dictated by culture and sensitivity data. As previously mentioned, all patients with cirrhosis and upper GI bleeding warrant antibiotic prophylaxis for spontaneous bacterial peritonitis (SBP). In cases of confirmed SBP, concurrent albumin administration (1.5 g/kg at time of diagnosis and 1 g/kg on day 3) reduces the incidence of renal impairment and death compared with antibiotics alone.[49]

Acute calculous cholecystitis is common among cirrhotic patients and maintaining a high suspicion for the disease is essential. Treatment with percutaneous transhepatic cholecystostomy followed by delayed laparoscopic cholecystectomy has been shown to be both safe and effective in this patient population.[50]

Rehabilitation

Patients with liver disease are not immune to the numerous consequences of intensive care, including the constellation of physical, cognitive, and mental health complications collectively referred to as post–intensive care syndrome. Prior studies targeting inpatient rehabilitation of liver transplant recipients have associated low albumin level and longer length of acute care stays with prolonged and less efficient rehabilitation periods.[51] This finding highlights the significance of minimizing sedation to enable early mobilization as well as aggressive weaning from support devices, including mechanical ventilation. Further, it is incumbent on all physicians involved in the care of patients with liver disease to have frequent and frank discussions regarding goals of care and code status.

SUMMARY

Caring for critically ill patients with acute and/or chronic liver dysfunction poses a unique challenge. Proper resuscitation and early consideration for transfer to liver transplant centers have resulted in improved outcomes. Liver support devices, including acellular models (Molecular Adsorbent Recirculating System [MARS] and the Prometheus system) and cellular models (Extracorporeal Liver Assist Device [ELAD] and the Nyberg device) have not yet shown mortality benefit, but they hold promise in the critical care of patients with liver disease.

REFERENCES

1. Fink MP, Hayes M, Soni N. Aphorism IV 60. Stephanus of Athens. Commentary on Hippocrates' aphorisms. Sections III – IV. Berlin: Akadamie Verlag. Classic papers in critical care. 2nd edition. London: Springer; 2008. p. 171.
2. Matuschak GM, Rinaldo JE. Organ interactions in the adult respiratory distress syndrome during sepsis. Role of the liver in host defense. Chest 1988;94(2): 400–6.
3. Bradfield JW. Control of spillover. The importance of Kupffer-cell function in clinical medicine. Lancet 1974;2(7885):883–6.
4. Bilzer M, Roggel F, Gerbes AL. Role of Kupffer cells in host defense and liver disease. Liver Int 2006;26(10):1175–86.
5. Wu Y, Ren J, Zhou B, et al. Laser speckle contrast imaging for measurement of hepatic microcirculation during the sepsis: a novel tool for early detection of microcirculation dysfunction. Microvasc Res 2015;97:137–46.
6. Morel J, Li JY, Eyenga P, et al. Early adverse changes in liver microvascular circulation during experimental septic shock are not linked to an absolute nitric oxide deficit. Microvasc Res 2013;90:187–91.
7. Kuhla A, Norden J, Abshagen K, et al. RAGE blockade and hepatic microcirculation in experimental endotoxaemic liver failure. Br J Surg 2013;100(9): 1229–39.
8. Mookerjee R. Acute-on-chronic liver failure: the liver and portal haemodynamics. Curr Opin Crit Care 2011;17(2):170–6.

9. McIntyre N. The limitations of conventional liver function tests. Semin Liver Dis 1983;3(4):265–74.

10. Doglio GR, Pusajo JF, Egurrola MA, et al. Gastric mucosal pH as a prognostic index of mortality in critically ill patients. Crit Care Med 1991;19(8):1037–40.

11. Gutierrez G, Palizas F, Doglio G, et al. Gastric intramucosal pH as a therapeutic index of tissue oxygenation in critically ill patients. Lancet 1992;339(8787): 195–9.

12. Maynard ND, Bihari DJ, Dalton RN, et al. Liver function and splanchnic ischemia in critically ill patients. Chest 1997;111(1):180–7.

13. Gys T, Hubens A, Neels H, et al. Prognostic value of gastric intramural pH in surgical intensive care patients. Crit Care Med 1988;16(12):1222–4.

14. Foreman MG, Mannino DM, Moss M. Cirrhosis as a risk factor for sepsis and death: analysis of the national hospital discharge survey. Chest 2003;124(3): 1016–20.

15. Kavli M, Strøm T, Carlsson M, et al. The outcome of critical illness in decompensated alcoholic liver cirrhosis. Acta Anaesthesiol Scand 2012;56(8):987–94.

16. Parkash O, Mumtaz K, Hamid S, et al. MELD score: utility and comparison with King's College criteria in non-acetaminophen acute liver failure. J Coll Physicians Surg Pak 2012;22(8):492–6.

17. Kamath PS, Wiesner RH, Malinchoc M, et al. A model to predict survival in patients with end-stage liver disease. Hepatology 2001;33(2):464–70.

18. Stravitz RT, Kramer DJ. Chapter 20-Acute liver failure. In: Sanyal, TD BMJ, editors. Zakim and Boyer's hepatology. 6th edition. St Louis (MO): WB Saunders; 2012. p. 327–51.

19. Vaquero J, Butterworth RF. Mechanisms of brain edema in acute liver failure and impact of novel therapeutic interventions. Neurol Res 2007;29(7):683–90.

20. Larsen FS, Wendon J. Prevention and management of brain edema in patients with acute liver failure. Liver Transpl 2008;14(Suppl 2):S90–6.

21. Dethloff TJ, Knudsen GM, Larsen FS. Cerebral blood flow autoregulation in experimental liver failure. J Cereb Blood Flow Metab 2008;28(5):916–26.

22. Blei AT, Olafsson S, Webster S, et al. Complications of intracranial pressure monitoring in fulminant hepatic failure. Lancet 1993;341(8838):157–8.

23. Bernal W, Hall C, Karvellas CJ, et al. Arterial ammonia and clinical risk factors for encephalopathy and intracranial hypertension in acute liver failure. Hepatology 2007;46(6):1844–52.

24. Larsen FS, Adel Hansen B, Pott F, et al. Dissociated cerebral vasoparalysis in acute liver failure. A hypothesis of gradual cerebral hyperaemia. J Hepatol 1996;25(2):145–51.

25. Aggarwal S, Kramer D, Yonas H, et al. Cerebral hemodynamic and metabolic changes in fulminant hepatic failure: a retrospective study. Hepatology 1994; 19(1):80–7.

26. Jalan R, Damink SW, Deutz NE, et al. Moderate hypothermia for uncontrolled intracranial hypertension in acute liver failure. Lancet 1999; 354(9185):1164–8.

27. Murphy N, Auzinger G, Bernel W, et al. The effect of hypertonic sodium chloride on intracranial pressure in patients with acute liver failure. Hepatology 2004; 39(2):464–70.

28. Lee WM, Larson AM, Stravitz RT. AASLD position paper: the management of acute liver failure: update 2011. The American Association for the Study of Liver Diseases. Alexandria (Virginia);2011.

29. Jones EA, Schafer DF, Ferenci P, et al. The GABA hypothesis of the pathogenesis of hepatic encephalopathy: current status. Yale J Biol Med 1984;57(3):301–16.

30. Murray JF, Dawson AM, Sherlock S. Circulatory changes in chronic liver disease. Am J Med 1958;24(3):358–67.

31. Bayley TJ, Segel N, Bishop JM. The circulatory changes in patients with cirrhosis of the liver at rest and during exercise. Clin Sci 1964;26:227–35.

32. Lobo DN, Awad S. Should chloride-rich crystalloids remain the mainstay of fluid resuscitation to prevent "pre-renal" acute kidney injury?: con. Kidney Int 2014; 86(6):1096–105.

33. Boniatti MM, Cardoso PRC, Castilho RK, et al. Is hyperchloremia associated with mortality in critically ill patients? A prospective cohort study. J Crit Care 2011; 26(2):175–9.

34. Eefsen M, Dethloff T, Frederiksen H-J, et al. Comparison of terlipressin and noradrenalin on cerebral perfusion, intracranial pressure and cerebral extracellular concentrations of lactate and pyruvate in patients with acute liver failure in need of inotropic support. J Hepatol 2007;47(3):381–6.

35. Spiess BD, Tuman KJ, McCarthy RJ, et al. Oxygen consumption and mixed venous oxygen saturation monitoring during orthotopic liver transplantation. J Clin Monit 1992;8(1):7–11.

36. Tapia P, Soto D, Bruhn A, et al. Impairment of exogenous lactate clearance in experimental hyperdynamic septic shock is not related to total liver hypoperfusion. Crit Care 2015;19(1):188.

37. Zampieri FG, Park M, Ranzani OT, et al. Anion gap corrected for albumin, phosphate and lactate is a good predictor of strong ion gap in critically ill patients: a nested cohort study. Rev Bras Ter Intensiva 2013;25(3):205–11.

38. Paramythiotis D, Kazamias P, Grosomanidis V, et al. Splanchnic ischemia during mechanical ventilation. Ann Gastroenterol 2008;21(1):45–52.

39. Matuschak GM, Rinaldo JE, Pinsky MR, et al. Effect of end-stage liver failure on the incidence and resolution of the adult respiratory distress syndrome. J Crit Care 1987;2(3):162–73.

40. Doyle HR, Marino IR, Miro A, et al. Adult respiratory distress syndrome secondary to end-stage liver disease—successful outcome following liver transplantation. Transplantation 1993;55(2):292–6.

41. Olson JC, Wendon J, Kramer DJ, et al. Intensive care of the patient with cirrhosis. Hepatology 2011;54(5):1864–72.

42. Bernal W, Auzinger G, Sizer E, et al. Intensive care management of acute liver failure. Semin Liver Dis 2008;28(2):188–200.

43. Jalan R, Gines P, Olson JC, et al. Acute-on chronic liver failure. J Hepatol 2012; 57(6):1336–48.

44. Thursz MR, Richardson P, Allison M, et al. Prednisolone or pentoxifylline for alcoholic hepatitis. N Engl J Med 2015;372(17):1619–28.

45. Mumtaz K, Azam Z, Hamid S, et al. Role of N-acetylcysteine in adults with non-acetaminophen-induced acute liver failure in a center without the facility of liver transplantation. Hepatol Int 2009;3(4):563–70.

46. Chavez-Tapia NC, Barrientos-Gutierrez T, Tellez-Avila FI, et al. Antibiotic prophylaxis for cirrhotic patients with upper gastrointestinal bleeding. Cochrane Database Syst Rev 2010;(9):CD002907.

47. Tsai M-H, Peng Y-S, Chen Y-C, et al. Adrenal insufficiency in patients with cirrhosis, severe sepsis and septic shock. Hepatology 2006;43(4):673–81.

48. Fernández J, Escorsell A, Zabalza M, et al. Adrenal insufficiency in patients with cirrhosis and septic shock: effect of treatment with hydrocortisone on survival. Hepatology 2006;44(5):1288–95.

49. Sort P, Navasa M, Arroyo V, et al. Effect of intravenous albumin on renal impairment and mortality in patients with cirrhosis and spontaneous bacterial peritonitis. N Engl J Med 1999;341(6):403–9.

50. Yao Z, Hu K, Huang P, et al. Delayed laparoscopic cholecystectomy is safe and effective for acute severe calculous cholecystitis in patients with advanced cirrhosis: a single center experience. Gastroenterol Res Pract 2014;2014: e178908.

51. Cortazzo MH, Helkowski W, Pippin B, et al. Acute inpatient rehabilitation of 55 patients after liver transplantation. Am J Phys Med Rehabil 2005;84(11):880–4.

Current Evidence for Extracorporeal Liver Support Systems in Acute Liver Failure and Acute-on-Chronic Liver Failure

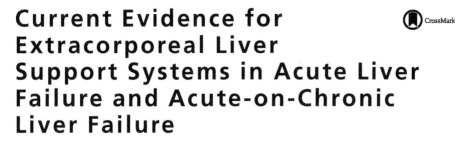

Constantine J. Karvellas, MD, SM, FRCPC[a,b,*],
Ram M. Subramanian, MD[c,d]

KEYWORDS

- Extracorporeal liver support • Albumin dialysis • Acute liver failure
- Acute-on-chronic liver failure • Extracorporeal liver assist device
- Liver transplantation

KEY POINTS

- Supporting detoxification and synthetic functions of the failing liver is the rationale for the use of extracorporeal liver support (ECLS) systems.
- Bioartificial ECLS (B-ECLS) systems incorporate a bioreactor containing various forms of hepatocytes to provide synthetic functions.
- Artificial and bioartificial liver support devices have shown certain detoxification capabilities and biochemical improvement in patients with acute liver failure (ALF) and acute-on-chronic liver failure (ACLF), but their effects have failed to correlate with survival benefit.
- High-volume plasmapheresis (HVP) is the only therapy that has demonstrated a statistically significant benefit in transplant-free survival in ALF patients.
- Further refinement of target populations and adequate endpoints, optimization of therapy delivery, and avoidance of futile therapy seem to be essential steps for future ECLS devices to become integrated in standard medical therapy (SMT) for specific subpopulations of ALF and ACLF patients.

Disclosure Statement: None.
[a] Division of Hepatology, University of Alberta, Edmonton, Alberta, Canada; [b] Division of Critical Care Medicine, University of Alberta, 1-40 Zeidler Ledcor Building, Edmonton, Alberta T6G-2X8, Canada; [c] Division of Hepatology, Emory University, Atlanta, GA, USA; [d] Division of Critical Care Medicine, Emory University, Atlanta, GA, USA
* Corresponding author. Liver Unit, Division of Gastroenterology, University of Alberta, 1-40 Zeidler Ledcor Building, Edmonton, Alberta T6G-2X8, Canada.
E-mail address: dean.karvellas@ualberta.ca

Crit Care Clin 32 (2016) 439–451
http://dx.doi.org/10.1016/j.ccc.2016.03.003
0749-0704/16/$ – see front matter © 2016 Elsevier Inc. All rights reserved.

INTRODUCTION: THE TWO SYNDROMES OF LIVER FAILURE
Acute Liver Failure

ALF is defined by hepatic encephalopathy (HE) and synthetic dysfunction within 26 weeks of the first symptoms of liver disease.[1] The most common cause of ALF in North America and Europe is acetaminophen (N-acetyl-p-aminophenol [APAP]).[2,3] Particularly in APAP-induced ALF, cerebral edema and intracranial hypertension continue to be major causes of morbidity and mortality along with multiorgan failure due to the systemic inflammatory response (SIRS).[4,5] Current management of ALF (in particular, hyperacute ALF) is directed at reducing intracranial hypertension, including osmotic agents (mannitol or hypertonic saline),[6] control of blood pressure, ammonia-lowering therapies (eg, hemofiltration[7]), and therapeutic hypothermia.[8]

Acute-on-Chronic Liver Failure

In contrast, ACLF is defined as patients with cirrhosis hospitalized for acute decompensation and organ failure who are at a high mortality risk.[9] ACLF usually presents as an acute deterioration in liver function over a 2-week to 4-week period in a patient with preexisting chronic liver disease. Similar to ALF, the lack of the metabolic and regulatory function of the liver results in life-threatening complications that may include variceal bleeding, acute kidney injury (AKI), HE, cardiovascular failure, and susceptibility to infections culminating in multiorgan failure.[10] Recently the chronic liver failure (CLIF)–sequential organ failure assessment (SOFA) score has demonstrated that accumulating organ failures in ACLF patients in the absence of transplant is associated with increased mortality.[9]

Rationale for Use of Extracorporeal Liver Support in Acute Liver Failure and Acute-on-Chronic Liver Failure

In both ALF and ACLF, toxins accumulate as a result of impaired hepatic function and clearance. Ammonia, inflammatory cytokines, aromatic amino acids, and endogenous benzodiazepines have been implicated in the development of HE and cerebral edema (ALF). Other systemic factors, such as nitric oxide and cytokines, have been linked with circulatory and renal dysfunction in liver failure. Proinflammatory cytokines and damage-associated molecular patterns (DAMPs) have broad effects, ranging from increased capillary permeability to modulating cell death and immune dysregulation.

Currently, the only definitive therapy for patients with ALF and ACLF when poor prognostic criteria are met is liver transplantation (LT). Many patients die, however, before a suitable graft is available and, for those who progress to multiorgan failure, LT is not an option. Particularly in APAP-ALF, however, the liver often maintains some regenerative capacity, so the rationale for supportive therapy and extracorporeal systems is to provide an environment facilitating recovery to create or prolong a window of opportunity for LT, or, in the best case scenario, until native liver recovery occurs in APAP-ALF without cerebral edema/multiorgan failure, or a period of stability for those with ACLF until an organ becomes available.[11]

From a theoretic perspective, an effective ECLS should assist 3 major hepatic functions: detoxification, biosynthesis, and regulation.

In both ALF and ACLF, aims of ECLS are to remove putative toxins, preventing further aggravation of liver failure; to stimulate liver regeneration; and to improve the pathophysiologic features of liver failure.[12] None of the devices currently available, however, fulfills these requirements completely.

EXTRACORPOREAL LIVER SUPPORT SYSTEMS: ARTIFICIAL AND BIOARTIFICIAL

ECLS systems that have been tested clinically belong to 1 of the following 2 categories:

1. Artificial ECLS systems are based on the principles of adsorption and filtration and are aimed at removing circulating toxins by using membranes with different pore sizes and adsorbent columns.
2. B-ECLS systems are hybrid devices that incorporate hepatocytes in a bioactive platform to improve the detoxification capacity and to support synthetic hepatic function.[13] Cells origins include human (including hepatoblastoma) and porcine.

ARTIFICIAL EXTRACORPOREAL LIVER SUPPORT: DETOXIFICATION AND THE ALBUMIN HYPOTHESIS

Albumin administration has been shown beneficial in spontaneous bacterial peritonitis and hepatorenal syndrome partly due to its ability to bind toxins.[14] Artificial ECLS technologies use albumin as a binding and scavenging molecule. Different albumin-based ECLS devices vary based on the following characteristics:

- Membrane types/porosity/selectivity
- Types of columns/filters
- Modality of renal replacement therapy used
- Need to have an albumin enriched dialysate
- Extracorporeal volume needed

Dialysis-related techniques include the Molecular Adsorbent Recirculating System (MARS [Teraklin AG, Rostock, Germany]) and single-pass albumin dialysis (SPAD).[15] These techniques involve dialyzing blood against an albumin-containing solution across a highly selective/small-porosity (<50 kDa) high-flux membrane. The blood-bound toxins are cleared by diffusion and taken up by the binding sites of the albumin dialysate. In contrast, plasma adsorption techniques, such as Prometheus (fractionated plasma separation and adsorption) (Fresenius, Hamburg, Germany) and HVP use more nonselective membranes (approximately 250 kDa) and do not use a parallel dialysate circuit.

Molecular Adsorbent Recirculating System

MARS was originally developed by Stange and colleagues[16] in 1993. The system consists of a blood circuit, an albumin circuit, and a classic renal circuit. Blood is dialyzed across an albumin-impregnated high-flux dialysis membrane; 600 mL of 20% human albumin in the albumin circuit acts as the dialysate. The albumin dialysate is subsequently cleansed via passage across 2 sequential adsorbent columns containing activated charcoal and anion exchange resin. These columns remove most of the water-soluble and albumin-bound toxins. Substances with a molecular weight of more than 50 kDa, such as essential hormones and growth factors bound to albumin, are not removed because of the small pore size of the membrane.[17]

Molecular Adsorbent Recirculating System and Acute-on-Chronic Liver Failure: Clinical Studies

In 2000, Mitzner and colleagues[18] reported 13 patients with ACLF and type 1 hepatorenal syndrome treated with MARS. Patients received a mean of 5 treatments and did not receive vasopressors nor were any transplanted. The investigators showed a 37.5% absolute survival benefit at day 7 versus 0% in controls. A significant decrease in creatinine and bilirubin was also noted in the MARS group.

Subsequently, Heemann and colleagues[19] randomized 23 patients with ACLF (19 were alcoholics) to MARS or SMT, including dialysis if necessary. Inclusion criteria included bilirubin greater than 340 μmol/L, HE greater than grade 2, and AKI. At day 30, 11 of 12 patients in the MARS group were still alive compared with only 6 of 11 in the control group ($P<.05$). There were also statistically significant decreases in bilirubin (43%) and bile acids (29%) in the MARS group but not in the control group. A statistically significant increase in mean arterial pressure (MAP) ($P<.05$) as well as reductions in creatinine and HE grade ($P<.06$) were noted in the MARS group.

In 2007, Hassanein and colleagues[20] published a randomized controlled study of 70 ACLF patients with grade 3 or grade 4 HE who received either MARS (n = 39) or SMT (n = 31). The need for ventilation and the use of sedation were equal in both groups. Patients in the MARS group received therapy for 6 hours daily for 5 days or until a 2-grade improvement in HE was achieved. In the MARS group, 34% achieved a 2-grade improvement in HE versus 19% in the SMT group ($P = .044$). This study was not powered to look at mortality.

The results of the largest randomized trial of the use of MARS in ACLF (RELIEF study [Therapeutic Impact of Albumin Dialysis With the Molecular Adsorbents Recirculating System (MARS®) in Severely Decompensated Chronic Liver Disease]) were reported by Banares and colleagues[21] in 2013. In this study, 189 patients with ACLF from 19 European centers were randomly assigned to receive either MARS plus SMT (n = 95) or SMT alone (n = 94). The main endpoint of the study was 28-day survival. Patients randomly assigned to the MARS arm received up to ten 6-hour to 8-hour sessions of MARS. Improvement of HE was also more frequent in the MARS arm (from grade II–IV to grade 0–I; 63% vs 38%; $P = .07$). There was no difference, however, in 28-day survival between the MARS and SMT groups either by intention-to-treat or per-protocol analysis (60. 7% vs 58.9% and 60% vs 59.2%, respectively). Adverse events were similar in both groups, a fact that has been observed across the different studies.

MOLECULAR ADSORBENT RECIRCULATING SYSTEM AND ACUTE LIVER FAILURE

In 2003, Schmidt and colleagues[22] conducted a study to assess the effects of a single 6-hour MARS treatment on hemodynamics, oxygen consumption, and biochemical profile in 13 ALF patients (APAP, n = 10) with HE grade III/IV. Eight received MARS therapy and 5 received SMT with cooling to match hypothermia induced by MARS. Systemic vascular resistance index increased by 46% in the MARS group during the 6-hour run treatment versus a 6% increase in the controls ($P<.0001$). MAP also increased in the MARS group ($P<.001$) whereas pressure was unchanged in controls. Compared with baseline, there were significant reductions in bilirubin, creatinine, and urea ($P<.05$) but not in ammonia in the MARS group. Survival was similar between groups. In a controlled study of 27 patients treated for ALF due to cardiogenic shock, El Banayosy and colleagues[23] demonstrated nonsignificant reductions in conjugated and total bilirubin and mortality (**Table 1**). It is unclear, however, whether this population truly met criteria for ALF, because there is no mention of grade of HE.

The most robust study of MARS in ALF was a recently published randomized, controlled trial performed in 16 French transplant centers (FULMAR [FULMAREfficacy and Safety of the Albumin Dialysis MARS Therapy in Patients With Fulminant and Sub-fulminant Hepatic Failure] study) by Saliba and colleagues.[27] This study compared the impact of MARS plus SMT versus SMT alone in patients with ALF fulfilling transplant criteria; 53 patients were randomized to receive MARS therapy whereas 49 had SMT.

Table 1
Artificial extracorporeal liver support in acute liver failure/acute-on-chronic liver failure

Study	N	Device	Biochemical	Cardiovascular System	Central Nervous System	Survival
ACLF						
Mitzner et al,[18] 2000	13	MARS	Yes	Yes	No	Yes (37.5% vs 0% at 7 d)
Heemann et al,[19] 2002	24	MARS	Yes	Yes	Yes	Yes (90% vs 55% at 30 d)
Sen et al,[24] 2004	18	MARS	Yes	No	Yes	No (45% in both)
Laleman et al,[25] 2006	18	MARS/Prometheus	Yes	No	N/A	N/A
Hassanein et al,[20] 2007	70	MARS	Yes	N/A	Yes	N/A
Kribben et al,[26] 2012	143	Prometheus	Yes	N/A	—	No effect on 28/90 d survival
Banares et al,[21] 2013	189	MARS	Yes	N/A	Yes	No effect on 28 d survival
ALF						
Schmidt et al,[22] 2003	13	MARS	Yes	Yes	N/A	No
El Banayosy et al,[23] 2004	27	MARS	No	N/A	N/A	Yes (50% vs 32%)[a]
Saliba et al,[27] 2013	102	MARS	Yes	N/A	N/A	No effect on survival
Larsen et al,[28] 2016	182	HVP	Yes	Yes	Yes	Yes

Biochemical improvements: statistically significant reduction in bilirubin, bile acids, creatinine, and ammonia.
Abbreviation: N/A, not assessed
[a] Patients may have had acute liver injury (ischemic hepatitis) and not ALF.

Overall, there were no significant differences in 6-month survival between the MARS (85%) versus SMT (76%) groups ($P = .28$). A major confounder, however, was that the median listing-to-transplant time was only 16.2 hours, and 75% of enrolled patients underwent transplant within 24 hours. In the MARS group, 14 of 53 patients did not complete at least 5 hours of MARS therapy prior to LT or death. Hence, although overall negative, this study may have been underpowered to show a potential benefit in 6-month transplant-free survival in APAP-ALF patients (MARS 85% vs SMT 68%; $P = .40$), a group with greater potential for hepatic recovery.

Molecular Adsorbent Recirculating System and Inflammatory Profile

Stadlbauer[31] assessed cytokine levels in 8 patients with ACLF of diverse causes undergoing alternating treatments with MARS and Prometheus in a random crossover design; 34 treatments (17 MARS and 17 Prometheus) were available for analysis. Although measurable plasma clearances were detected for interleukin (IL)-6, IL-8, IL-10, and tumor necrosis factor (TNF)-α, none was significant for MARS or Prometheus. Based on these studies, MARS does not seem to have a significant impact on the inflammatory profile in ACLF.

Single-Pass Albumin Dialysis

SPAD differs from MARS in that it uses a standard continuous renal replacement therapy system without any additional columns or circuits. Blood is dialyzed against a standard dialysis solution with the addition of 4.4% albumin in the dialysate. SPAD has been evaluated in a case-control fashion in APAP-ALF but failed to show biochemical or mortality improvements.[32]

Prometheus: Fractionated Plasma Separation and Adsorption

Prometheus, or fractionated plasma separation and adsorption, was initially introduced in 1999. In this circuit, patient plasma is fractionated through an albumin-permeable filter with a cutoff of 250 kDa. Albumin and other plasma proteins cross the membrane and pass across 2 columns in series: 1 an anion-exchange column and another a neutral resin adsorber. The cleansed albumin/plasma is returned to the standard blood pool circuit where it is then treated by conventional high-flux hemodialysis.

To date there have been few significant controlled studies examining the impact of Prometheus; both studies examined ACLF patients only. Laleman and colleagues[25] compared the hemodynamic effects of Prometheus with MARS in 18 patients with ACLF secondary to severe alcoholic hepatitis (Maddrey score >60): 6 patients received MARS, 6 received Prometheus, and 6 received SMT (including renal replacement therapy). After 3 consecutive days of therapy (mean approximately 6 hours), both MARS and Prometheus reduced serum bilirubin ($P<.005$); MARS increased MAP (Δ +9 mm Hg; $P<.05$) and systemic vascular resistance index (Δ +220 dynes/cm^5/m^2; $P<.05$) compared with Prometheus. No difference in hemodynamics was noted between Prometheus and SMT. Levels of endogenous norepinephrine, aldosterone, and vasopressin were reduced ($P<.05$) in the MARS group, although there was no statistically significant change in the Prometheus or SMT arms.

In 2012, Kribben and colleagues[26] reported the HELIOS (Effects of fractionated plasma separation and adsorption on survival in patients with acute-on-chronic liver failure) trial, a prospective study of 145 ACLF patients who were randomly assigned to receive Prometheus plus SMT versus SMT alone. Primary endpoints of the study were the probability of survival at days 28 and 90, irrespective of LT. Both groups were similar at the baseline. Serum bilirubin levels decreased significantly in patients randomly assigned to receive fractionated plasma separation and adsorption compared with the group receiving SMT alone. In an intention-to-treat analysis, the 28-day survival was similar between Prometheus (66%) and SMT (63%) groups (P = .70) as was 90-day survival (Prometheus 47% vs SMT38%; P = .35). Baseline factors independently associated with poor prognosis were a high SOFA score, gastrointestinal bleeding, spontaneous bacterial peritonitis, AKI, and the combination of alcoholic and viral etiologies of liver disease. Similar to RELIEF (MARS), HELIOS may have suffered from confounding by indication; ACLF patients who were candidates for LT potentially have a different natural history from ACLF patients who were not LT candidates.

High-Volume Plasmapheresis

HVP with fresh frozen plasma is an established therapy used for immunologically driven disorders. Case series of HVP in patients with ALF have been shown to be safe,[33,34] to decrease the severity of HE, and to decrease vasopressor requirements.[35,36] Recently, Larsen and colleagues[28] published the first artificial ECLS study in ALF patients to demonstrate a statistically significant benefit in transplant-free survival using HVP. They prospectively randomized 183 ALF patients (1998–2010) in 3 European centers, of whom 91 patients received SMT and 92 received HVP above and beyond SMT. HVP was defined as 15% of ideal body weight (8–12 L of fresh frozen plasma), with individual runs lasting approximately 9 hours per treatment. Patients received a mean of 2.4 therapies, with only 1 patient in the HVP arm not receiving the therapy due to early LT. In an intention-to-treat analysis, survival to hospital discharge was 58.7% for patients treated with HVP versus 47.8% for the patients who received SMT alone (hazard ratio for HVP vs SMT with stratification for LT 0.56; 95% CI, 0.36–0.86; P = .0083). Biochemical markers (international normalized ratio, bilirubin, and ammonia) improved significantly in the HVP group compared with controls. Furthermore, in a nested cohort study of a subset of 30 ALF patients, patients undergoing HVP had significantly reduced circulating levels of DAMPs, including circulating histone-associated DNA), TNF-α, and IL-6. Furthermore, phenotypic markers of monocyte activation neutrophil activation (IL-8 expression) were downmodulated, suggesting that HVP suppresses the SIRS associated with ALF.

ARTIFICIAL EXTRACORPOREAL LIVER SUPPORT: ADVERSE EFFECT PROFILE

Hemostasis is the result of a complex interaction between procoagulant, anticoagulant, and fibrinolytic proteins, many of which may be affected by liver failure and, furthermore, ECLS.[37] Theoretically, less selective systems, such as Prometheus, potentially are at a higher risk than MARS due to the larger pore size of filters used. Furthermore, some artificial ECLS circuits require heparin[38] or citrate for anticoagulation.[39] Faybik and colleagues[40] described 33 patients undergoing 61 MARS treatments (15 with ALF, 15 with ACLF, and 3 with allograft dysfunction post-transplant). Although there was a statistically significant decrease in platelets and fibrinogen, platelet function as measured by thromboelastography was unaffected. Nonetheless, larger randomized controlled studies of MARS, Prometheus, and HVP in ALF and ACLF have not shown a significant increase in adverse events, including bleeding, over SMT.[21,26–28]

Bioartificial Extracorporeal Liver Support: Design

In theory, B-ECLS platforms could have advantages over artificial ECLS by providing synthetic replacement as well as detoxification functionality, particularly in APAP-ALF, where this is significant potential for hepatic recovery. They require a cell source that has been traditionally been derived from human or porcine hepatocytes. What has limited their widespread evaluation and adoption, however, have been their complex nature, necessity for a critical bioactive mass, more complex cumbersome technology, cost, and, in cases where porcine hepatocytes cell lines have been used, the risk of xenotransmission. To date, a vast majority of studies that have assessed the applicability and efficacy of B-ECLS in ALF and ACLF have included small numbers of patients and been uncontrolled. To date, 2 devices have been evaluated in detail: Extracorporeal Liver Assist Device (ELAD, Vital Therapies Inc, San Diego, USA) and HepatAssist (Arbios, USA).

Bioartificial Extracorporeal Liver Support in Acute Liver Failure

ELAD is based on a platform of human-derived hepatocytes. It has been evaluated in ALF by Ellis and colleagues[29] in 24 patients, of whom 7 met poor prognostic criteria. Patients were evenly randomized to ELAD plus SMT versus SMT. Patients were stratified by the absence (group I, n = 17 patients) or presence (group II, n = 7 patients) of meeting poor prognostic criteria. There were no differences, however, in survival in the low-risk (78% vs 75% in group I) or high-risk (33% vs 25% in group II) groups (Table 2).[29]

More recently, a randomized controlled trial of ELAD therapy in the treatment of severe alcoholic hepatitis has been concluded, and the results have been published in abstract form.[41] In this study (VTI-208 [Assess Safety and Efficacy of ELAD (Extracorporeal Liver Assist System) in Subjects With Alcohol-Induced Liver Failure]), 203 patients with severe alcoholic hepatitis (defined as a Maddrey discriminant function >32) and a Model for End-Stage Liver Disease (MELD) score less than or equal to 35, were randomized to 3 to 5 days of ELAD therapy (n = 96) or SMT (n = 107). The primary endpoint of the study was overall survival up to 91 days. In an intention-to-treat analysis, there was no significant difference in survival (52.1% vs 52.3%; hazard ratio 1.027; P = .9). In a predefined subgroup of patients with a MELD less than 28 (n = 120), however, ELAD was associated with a trend toward higher overall survival to 91 days (71% vs 57%, P = .077). Based on this subgroup analysis that is hypothesis generating, a subsequent study is planned that is designed to assess the efficacy of ELAD in a less sick population of alcoholic hepatitis patients.

HepatAssist incorporates porcine-purified hepatocytes in a bioreactor and has been evaluated in a large-scale, randomized, multicenter clinical trial. Demetriou and colleagues[30] randomly assigned 171 patients with ALF or with primary nonfunction after LT that were randomly assigned to receive SMT or SMT plus support with the

Table 2
Evidence for bioartificial extracorporeal liver support in acute liver failure/acute-on-chronic liver failure

Study	N	Device	Cell Type	Survival
ACLF				
VTI-208 2015	203	ELAD	Human (cultured C3A)	No (90 d 59 vs 62%; P = .74)
ALF				
Ellis et al,[29] 1996	24	ELAD	Human (Cultured C3A)	No difference in survival
Demetriou et al,[30] 2004	171	HepatAssist	Porcine (Cryopreserved)	No (30 d 71% vs 62%; P = .26)

Biochemical improvements: statistically significant reduction in bilirubin, bile acids, creatinine, and ammonia.

HepatAssist system. The primary endpoint of the study was 30-day survival (with or without LT) and adjusted by confounding factors in a multivariate model. The number of HepatAssist treatments ranged from 1 to 9 (mean, 2.9) per patient. Overall, 30-day survival was similar in groups in the entire cohort (HepatAssist 71% vs SMT 62%; $P = .26$) as well as after excluding primary nonfunction patients ($P = .12$). The trial was prematurely stopped because of futility in the predetermined safety interim analysis.

Is It Wise to Pool Extracorporeal Liver Support Data in Meta-analysis for Acute Liver Failure or Acute-on-Chronic Liver Failure Patients?

Due to the volume of underpowered studies, theoretically meta-analysis/metaregression could aid in determine if ECLS has added merit not defined in individual studies. Several systematic reviews and meta-analyses, however, have been published in recent years with heterogeneous results. Kjaergard and colleagues[42] pooled data for ECLS (both artificial and bioartificial) separately for ALF and ACLF from 12 randomized trials. Compared with SMT, ECLS had a significant beneficial effect on HE (relative risk [RR] 0.67; 95% CI, 0.52–0.86), but they had no significant effects on mortality (RR 0.86; 95% CI, 0.65–1.12). Meta-regression analysis indicated that the effect of liver support systems depended on the type of liver failure; ECLS seemed to reduce mortality by 33% in ACLF (RR 0.67; 95% CI, 0.51–0.90) but not in ALF (RR 0.95; 95% CI, 0.71–1.29). In contrast, the meta-analysis by Stutchfield and colleagues[43,44] concluded that ECLS (both artificial and bioartificial) significantly improved survival in ALF (RR 0.70; $P = .05$) but not in ACLF (RR 0.87; P 5 .37). Finally, the most recent meta-analysis, which included studies from 1973 to 2012, found a decrease in mortality in patients with ACLF patients treated with artificial ECLS (RR 0.80; 95% CI, 0.66–0.96; $P = .018$) and in patients with ALF treated with B-ECLS (RR 0.69; 95% CI, 0.50–0.94; $P = .018$).[43] These conflicting results from these meta-analysis suggest significant confounding/bias from observational studies included. Given the heterogeneity in these trials in follow-up period, etiology of ALF/ACLF and severity of illness/organ failure, divergent results/conclusions are hardly surprising. Given that none of these studies included recent large MARS (RELIEF and FULMAR) or HVP studies, none of these studies likely answers questions raised from individual trials.

DISCUSSION: FUTURE DIRECTIONS

There continues to be great interest and potential for ECLS. At present it is difficult to make an evidence-based recommendation supporting artificial ECLS. Of this group, MARS is the best-studied albumin dialysis technology in ALF and ACLF. Although studies have consistently demonstrated biochemical improvement and improvement in HE with MARS,[20] recent large randomized studies in ACLF (RELIEF)[21] and ALF (FULMAR)[27] showed no survival benefit. The HELIOS study examining Prometheus in ACLF was also disappointing.[26] These studies shared some common methodological limitations in study design. Within studies in ALF and ACLF, heterogeneous groups of patients with varying causes with different natural histories were often lumped together. Several studies did not stratify patients based on severity of illness (eg, MELD, CLIF-SOFA); hence, it is difficult to assess patient matching and, furthermore, the impact of underlying disease on patient mortality with or without treatment. Furthermore due to cointerventions, such as LT, not all patients received prespecified durations of ECLS therapy. When examining RELIEF AND HELIOS, it may have been more parsimonious to examine only ACLF patients who were candidates for LT because ACLF patients with multiorgan failure portends poor outcomes.[9] Successfully bridging patients to LT may warrant further consideration because the primary endpoint over a 30-day to 90-day survival.

In ALF, it may be wise to focus future studies on APAP-induced ALF patients because they have the highest chance of spontaneous recovery of hepatic function and ECLS potentially has a role even in patients who are not candidates for LT (psychosocial and medical contraindications) as a bridge to recovery. The FULMAR study was underpowered to evaluate this subgroup but this was the only subgroup with a potential mortality difference.[27] One explanation for this is that the predominant mechanism responsible for the development of cerebral edema/multiorgan failure in hyperacute ALF is activation of and release of proinflammatory cytokines DAMPs as a result of massive hepatocyte necrosis.[47] In the only artificial ECLS study to show a benefit in transplant-free survival, Larsen and colleagues[28] demonstrated in ALF patients undergoing HVP that patients in the HVP group had significantly reduced circulating levels of DAMPs and proinflammatory cytokines with concomitant decrease in neutrophil activation. Dampening of the SIRS cascade was also consistent with the observed improvement in evidence of multiorgan failure as measured by SOFA and CLIF-SOFA. Given that APAP-ALF patients present early with multiorgan failure and up-regulated SIRS response, studies of future artificial and B-ECLS devices should consider their impact on the proinflammatory cascade, especially in APAP-ALF.

Although it is clear that current artificial and B-ECLS devices have limitations, potentially the greatest area for future research is in the improvement/refinement of bioartificial platforms. To date, studies of ELAD (human-derived hepatocytes) and HepatAssist (porcine hepatocytes) have been disappointing.[29,30] Further research into other functional cell sources (genetically modified liver cell lines, humanized pig cells, and hepatocyte spheroids) is ongoing.[45,46] Future studies will likely have to weigh the added levels of complexity and expense compared with purely detoxifying systems, such as HVP.

Irrespective of advances in technologies, future studies will need to avoid the methodological pitfalls of the past. Target patient populations should be homogenous with respect to causes (eg, APAP-ALF) or natural history (eg, only ACLF patients listed for LT). Patients enrolled into future trials should be comparable with respect to severity of illness (eg, number of organ failures and CLIF-SOFA) are target subpopulations need to be delineated further to avoid futile therapy. Other concomitant therapies (mechanical ventilation, antibiotics, and renal replacement therapy) will need to be consistent so that outcomes are not impacted by cointerventions.

REFERENCES

1. O'Grady JG, Williams R. Classification of acute liver failure. Lancet 1993;342:743.
2. Fagan E, Wannan G. Reducing paracetamol overdoses. BMJ 1996;313:1417–8.
3. Larson AM, Polson J, Fontana RJ, et al. Acetaminophen-induced acute liver failure: results of a United States multicenter, prospective study. Hepatology 2005; 42:1364–72.
4. Ware AJ, D'Agostino AN, Combes B. Cerebral edema: a major complication of massive hepatic necrosis. Gastroenterology 1971;61:877–84.
5. Bernal W, Wendon J. Acute liver failure; clinical features and management. Eur J Gastroenterol Hepatol 1999;11:977–84.
6. Murphy N, Auzinger G, Bernel W, et al. The effect of hypertonic sodium chloride on intracranial pressure in patients with acute liver failure. Hepatology 2004;39: 464–70.

7. Slack AJ, Auzinger G, Willars C, et al. Ammonia clearance with haemofiltration in adults with liver disease. Liver Int 2014;34:42–8.
8. Jalan R, Olde Damink SW, Deutz NE, et al. Moderate hypothermia in patients with acute liver failure and uncontrolled intracranial hypertension. Gastroenterology 2004;127:1338–46.
9. Moreau R, Jalan R, Gines P, et al. Acute-on-chronic liver failure is a distinct syndrome that develops in patients with acute decompensation of cirrhosis. Gastroenterology 2013;144:1426–37, 37.e1–9.
10. Sen S, Williams R, Jalan R. The pathophysiological basis of acute-on-chronic liver failure. Liver 2002;22(Suppl 2):5–13.
11. Sen S, Williams R, Jalan R. Emerging indications for albumin dialysis. Am J Gastroenterol 2005;100:468–75.
12. Nyberg SL. Bridging the gap: advances in artificial liver support. Liver Transpl 2012;18(Suppl 2):S10–4.
13. Allen JW, Hassanein T, Bhatia SN. Advances in bioartificial liver devices. Hepatology 2001;34:447–55.
14. Evans TW. Review article: albumin as a drug–biological effects of albumin unrelated to oncotic pressure. Aliment Pharmacol Ther 2002;16(Suppl 5):6–11.
15. Mitzner S, Klammt S, Stange J, et al. Albumin regeneration in liver support-comparison of different methods. Ther Apher Dial 2006;10:108–17.
16. Stange J, Ramlow W, Mitzner S, et al. Dialysis against a recycled albumin solution enables the removal of albumin-bound toxins. Artif Organs 1993;17:809–13.
17. Stange J, Mitzner SR, Risler T, et al. Molecular adsorbent recycling system (MARS): clinical results of a new membrane-based blood purification system for bioartificial liver support. Artif Organs 1999;23:319–30.
18. Mitzner SR, Stange J, Klammt S, et al. Improvement of hepatorenal syndrome with extracorporeal albumin dialysis MARS: results of a prospective, randomized, controlled clinical trial. Liver Transpl 2000;6:277–86.
19. Heemann U, Treichel U, Loock J, et al. Albumin dialysis in cirrhosis with superimposed acute liver injury: a prospective, controlled study. Hepatology 2002;36:949–58.
20. Hassanein TI, Tofteng F, Brown RS Jr, et al. Randomized controlled study of extracorporeal albumin dialysis for hepatic encephalopathy in advanced cirrhosis. Hepatology 2007;46:1853–62.
21. Banares R, Nevens F, Larsen FS, et al. Extracorporeal albumin dialysis with the molecular adsorbent recirculating system in acute-on-chronic liver failure: the RELIEF trial. Hepatology 2013;57:1153–62.
22. Schmidt LE, Wang LP, Hansen BA, et al. Systemic hemodynamic effects of treatment with the molecular adsorbents recirculating system in patients with hyperacute liver failure: a prospective controlled trial. Liver Transpl 2003;9:290–7.
23. El Banayosy A, Kizner L, Schueler V, et al. First use of the Molecular adsorbent recirculating system technique on patients with hypoxic liver failure after cardiogenic shock. ASAIO J 2004;50:332–7.
24. Sen S, Davies NA, Mookerjee RP, et al. Pathophysiological effects of albumin dialysis in acute-on-chronic liver failure: a randomized controlled study. Liver Transpl 2004;10:1109–19.
25. Laleman W, Wilmer A, Evenepoel P, et al. Effect of the molecular adsorbent recirculating system and Prometheus devices on systemic haemodynamics and vasoactive agents in patients with acute-on-chronic alcoholic liver failure. Crit Care 2006;10:R108.

26. Kribben A, Gerken G, Haag S, et al. Effects of fractionated plasma separation and adsorption on survival in patients with acute-on-chronic liver failure. Gastroenterology 2012;142:782–9.e3.

27. Saliba F, Camus C, Durand F, et al. Albumin dialysis with a noncell artificial liver support device in patients with acute liver failure: a randomized, controlled trial. Ann Intern Med 2013;159:522–31.

28. Larsen FS, Schmidt LE, Bernsmeier C, et al. High-volume plasma exchange in patients with acute liver failure: an open randomised controlled trial. J Hepatol 2016;64(1):69–78.

29. Ellis AJ, Hughes RD, Wendon JA, et al. Pilot-controlled trial of the extracorporeal liver assist device in acute liver failure. Hepatology 1996;24:1446–51.

30. Demetriou AA, Brown RS Jr, Busuttil RW, et al. Prospective, randomized, multi-center, controlled trial of a bioartificial liver in treating acute liver failure. Ann Surg 2004;239:660–7 [discussion: 667–70].

31. Stadlbauer V. Effect of extracorporeal liver suppor by MARS and Prometheus on serum cytokines in acute-on-chronic liver failure (AoCLF). Crit Care 2006; 10:1–20.

32. Karvellas CJ, Bagshaw SM, McDermid RC, et al. A case-control study of single-pass albumin dialysis for acetaminophen-induced acute liver failure. Blood Purif 2009;28:151–8.

33. Kondrup J, Almdal T, Vilstrup H, et al. High volume plasma exchange in fulminant hepatic failure. Int J Artif Organs 1992;15:669–76.

34. Nakamura T, Ushiyama C, Suzuki S, et al. Effect of plasma exchange on serum tissue inhibitor of metalloproteinase 1 and cytokine concentrations in patients with fulminant hepatitis. Blood Purif 2000;18:50–4.

35. Larsen FS, Ejlersen E, Hansen BA, et al. Systemic vascular resistance during high-volume plasmapheresis in patients with fulminant hepatic failure: relationship with oxygen consumption. Eur J Gastroenterol Hepatol 1995;7: 887–92.

36. Larsen FS, Hansen BA, Ejlersen E, et al. Cerebral blood flow, oxygen metabolism and transcranial Doppler sonography during high-volume plasmapheresis in fulminant hepatic failure. Eur J Gastroenterol Hepatol 1996;8:261–5.

37. Doria C, Mandalà L, Smith JD, et al. Thromboelastography used to assess coagulation during treatment with molecular adsorbent recirculating system. Clin Transplant 2004;18:365–71.

38. Tan HK, Yang WS, Chow P, et al. Anticoagulation minimization is safe and effective in albumin liver dialysis using the molecular adsorbent recirculating system. Artif Organs 2007;31:193–9.

39. Meijers B, Laleman W, Vermeersch P, et al. A prospective randomized open-label crossover trial of regional citrate anticoagulation vs. anticoagulation free liver dialysis by the Molecular Adsorbents Recirculating System. Crit Care 2012;16:R20.

40. Faybik P, Bacher A, Kozek-Langenecker SA, et al. Molecular adsorbent recirculating system and hemostasis in patients at high risk of bleeding: an observational study. Crit Care 2006;10:R24.

41. Thompson JA, Subramanian R, Al-Khafaji A, et al. The effect of extracorporeal C3a Cellular therapy in severe alcoholic hepatitis- the Elad trial. Hepatology 2015;62(6 Suppl) [Abstract # LB-1; 1379A].

42. Kjaergard LL, Liu J, Als-Nielsen B, et al. Artificial and bioartificial support systems for acute and acute-on-chronic liver failure: a systematic review. JAMA 2003;289: 217–22.

43. Stutchfield BM, Simpson K, Wigmore SJ. Systematic review and meta-analysis of survival following extracorporeal liver support. Br J Surg 2011;98:623–31.
44. Zheng Z, Li X, Li Z, et al. Artificial and bioartificial liver support systems for acute and acute-on-chronic hepatic failure: a meta-analysis and meta-regression. Exp Ther Med 2013;6:929–36.
45. Glorioso JM, van Wenum M, Chamuleau RA, et al. Pivotal preclinical trial of the spheroid reservoir bioartificial liver. J Hepatol 2015;63:388–98.
46. Lee KC, Baker LA, Stanzani G, et al. Extracorporeal liver assist device to exchange albumin and remove endotoxin in acute liver failure: results of a pivotal pre-clinical study. J Hepatol 2015;63:634–42.
47. Antoniades CG, Berry PA, Wendon JA, et al. The importance of immune dysfunction in determining outcome in acute liver failure. J Hepatol 2008;49:845–61.

Perioperative Care of the Liver Transplant Patient

Mark T. Keegan, MB, MRCPI, MSc[a],*, David J. Kramer, MD[b,c]

KEYWORDS

- Liver transplantation • Intensive care • Postoperative • Mechanical ventilation
- Complications • Anesthesia

KEY POINTS

- Liver transplantation is a major undertaking that requires a multidisciplinary team. Communication between the intensivist and other team members is essential.
- The transplant procedure is usually divided into pre-anhepatic, anhepatic, reperfusion, and neohepatic phases, each associated with specific anesthetic and surgical considerations.
- Although specific institutional practices may differ, anesthetic management requires anticipation of and response to hemodynamic derangements, provision for massive transfusion, and optimization of the patient for rapid recovery after the procedure.
- Although in some patients the transplant procedure itself is a brief interlude in a long intensive care unit (ICU) stay, in "routine" cases recipients spend a relatively brief time in the ICU postoperatively.
- Many aspects of postoperative care of the liver transplant recipient are predictable and suitable for implementation of management protocols and clinical pathways.

INTRODUCTION

Although the fundamentals remain the same, the perioperative care of the liver transplant (LT) recipient has changed significantly over the past 3 decades. Undoubtedly, LT surgery remains a major undertaking for the surgical and anesthesia teams, posing intellectual and physical challenges. With the evolution of surgical and anesthetic techniques, however, the procedure is now "routine," allowing for modifications of practice to decrease perioperative complications and costs. Living donor liver transplantation has allowed transplantation when recipients are optimized. The move toward "fast tracking" has shortened postoperative intensive care unit (ICU) length

Conflict of Interest Statement: Neither author has a commercial or financial conflict of interest relating to this article.
[a] Division of Critical Care, Department of Anesthesiology, Mayo Clinic, Charlton 1145, 200 1st Street Southwest, Rochester, MN 55905, USA; [b] Aurora Critical Care Service, 2901 W Kinnickinnic River Parkway, Milwaukee, WI 53215, USA; [c] University of Wisconsin, School of Medicine and Public Health, 750, Highland Avenue, Madison, WI 53705, USA
* Corresponding author.
E-mail address: keegan.mark@mayo.edu

Crit Care Clin 32 (2016) 453–473
http://dx.doi.org/10.1016/j.ccc.2016.02.005
0749-0704/16/$ – see front matter © 2016 Elsevier Inc. All rights reserved.

of stay or eliminated the need for ICU care altogether. In contrast to the opportunity to decrease ICU resource use afforded by these developments, however, further evolution is occurring. In the era of donor organ allocation according to Model for End Stage Liver Disease score, increasing numbers of patients are presenting for LT with established multiple organ failure and presenting to the operating room (OR) from the ICU rather than the general ward or outpatient area.[1-3] For such patients, the OR experience is a relatively brief time between 2 ICU stays. This article discusses the intraoperative management and early postoperative ICU care both of patients undergoing a "straightforward" LT and those for whom a preoperative requirement for intensive care complicates perioperative management.

INTRAOPERATIVE MANAGEMENT
Personnel

Institutional details vary, but in the United States key personnel involved in the operative procedure may be divided into 3 main groups. The surgical team includes the principal surgeon, usually at least 1 surgical assistant, a scrub nurse, and a circulating nurse. The anesthesia team usually includes an anesthesiologist aided by a nurse anesthetist or anesthesia resident or fellow. In many institutions, both surgical and anesthesia personnel are part of a dedicated LT call team. The third group includes a variety of essential personnel including transfusion medicine ("blood bank" and "autotransfusion") and clinical laboratory staff. Added to these, of course, are multiple other personnel who may be involved perioperatively, including members of nursing, pharmacy, radiology, respiratory therapy, clinical monitoring, and nephrology teams.[4] Intensivists are often integrated with the surgical or anesthesia teams and participate in candidate evaluation, particularly for those critically ill at the time of LT, and provide postoperative critical care.

Phases of the Liver Transplantation Procedure

The operative LT procedure has been traditionally divided into 3 phases, with reperfusion of the allograft liver as the event that distinguishes the anhepatic from the neohepatic (aka post-anhepatic) phase. **Table 1** details the phases of the procedure and the associated features.[5-7]

Key aspects of the donor and surgical procedure should be communicated to the team managing patients after the LT. Donor issues include the age of the donor, type of donor (donation after brain death [DBD], or donation after cardiac death [DCD]), cold ischemia time and warm ischemia time if DCD, and percentage of macrosteatosis in the allograft. Intraoperative issues include the duration of the procedure, units of blood products transfused, intraoperative anesthetic or surgical difficulties, warm ischemia time, and vascular and biliary anatomy.

Anesthesia Technique

General anesthesia with a tracheal tube in situ is the norm. The agents used for induction and maintenance of anesthesia are carefully chosen to provide anesthesia, amnesia, analgesia, and excellent surgical operating conditions while at the same time minimizing end-organ compromise.[5-7] Specific drugs and the doses used should be chosen with a view to allowing rapid emergence from anesthesia at the end of the case.[8] In the OR, after pre-medication with midazolam and fentanyl, induction is usually achieved with intravenous propofol. Alternatives include etomidate and ketamine. The risks of hemodynamic derangement associated with rapid sequence induction and intubation must be weighed against those of aspiration. A "balanced"

Table 1
Phases of the liver transplant procedure with associated features

Phase	Pre-anhepatic	Anhepatic	Reperfusion	Neohepatic
Timing	From incision to isolation of native liver from circulation	From isolation of native liver from circulation to reperfusion	A brief event at which the new liver is introduced into the patient's circulation	From reperfusion to the end of the procedure
Features	• Anesthesia induction • Line placement, skin incision • Dissection to allow removal of diseased liver • Obvious and insidious blood losses • Fluid shifts • Potential compression of native vessels during dissection • Worsening of preexisting coagulopathy	• Isolation of native liver from circulation • Removal of diseased liver • Implantation of new liver • Decrease in venous return (degree dependent on technique; modern "piggyback technique" affects venous return less than complete inferior vena cava occlusion technique) • Progressive coagulopathy • Progressive metabolic acidosis • Hypocalcemia	• Introduction of new liver into the circulation • Time of most instability • Potassium load, cytokine load, emboli, cold fluid • Hypotension common • Intracranial pressure may rise • Pulmonary hypertension may worsen • Arrhythmias • Coagulopathy may worsen	• From reperfusion to end of procedure • Reconstruction of hepatic artery • Construction of biliary anastomoses • New liver begins to function • Hemostasis • Continuing correction of coagulopathy, metabolic and acid base disorders • Optimization of cardiovascular parameters • Preparation for emergence

anesthetic technique is typically used for maintenance employing intravenous opiates (usually fentanyl at <20 μg/kg total for the case), and neuromuscular antagonists (usually atracurium or cisatracurium, which do not rely on the liver for metabolism) in combination with a volatile anesthetic agent (typically isoflurane or sevoflurane). In certain circumstances (eg, acute liver failure [ALF], in which intracranial hypertension exits) a total intravenous anesthetic is used and a continuous propofol infusion is administered instead of the volatile agent.[9–12]

Vascular Access, Monitors, and Other Considerations

Multiple vascular access devices are required for the transplantation procedure and are usually placed after induction, although some or all may be placed before induction, depending on the condition of the patient and institutional practice. One or more large-bore peripheral venous catheters (eg, "trauma catheter") should be placed for rapid transfusion of fluids and blood products and connected to a mechanical rapid infusion pump. Such devices usually have a reservoir to allow multiple products to be administered simultaneously while allowing high flows, bolus administration, warming, and debris/air filtering. Two arterial catheters are placed, one (usually brachial, occasionally femoral) to allow for reliable continuous blood pressure monitoring and the other (usually radial) to allow for blood sampling for laboratory analyses. The internal jugular vein is typically cannulated to allow placement of a large-bore introducer and a pulmonary artery catheter (PAC), often with a continuous oximetry feature. An additional large-bore catheter may be placed centrally if peripheral access is suboptimal or if veno-venous bypass (less commonly used now) is planned. Transesophageal echocardiography (TEE) is increasingly used as an adjunct, and in some centers TEE or continuous cardiac output monitors have replaced the use of PACs. Upper and lower warming blankets are placed in an effort to maintain normothermia. Norepinephrine is commonly administered to counteract volatile anesthetic–induced vasodilation in patients who already have decreased systemic vascular resistance because of their liver disease. A balanced electrolyte solution, preferably not buffered with lactate (eg, Plasmalyte) is administered as maintenance fluid. Administration of albumin affords resuscitation with less total volume because of its oncotic effects.

LT programs could not function successfully without reliable and efficient transfusion medicine support. Although transfusion requirements have decreased over time, allowing a decrease in the standard surgical blood order, the need for massive transfusion is still quite common.[13] Autotransfusion ("cell saver") is used routinely except for cases in which malignancy or infection is present. Massive transfusion may be required with the potential for dilutional coagulopathy, hyperkalemia, citrate intoxication leading to hypocalcemia, and hypothermia. Multiple measurements of complete blood count, electrolytes, glucose, arterial blood gases (ABGs), and coagulation parameters are required intraoperatively and this requires the availability of a clinical chemistry laboratory with a short reporting time.

IMMEDIATE POSTOPERATIVE CARE

In most centers, at the completion of the LT, the patient is transferred directly, still intubated, to the ICU.[14] Initial assessment is similar to the evaluation performed in the ICU after any major abdominal surgical procedure and will include consideration of the following:

- Hemodynamics: Labile hemodynamics reflect sequestration of fluid within the operative field and arterial vasodilation typical of liver disease. Recipients may require vasopressors but often require volume resuscitation. Crystalloid may be used judiciously but albumin allows resuscitation with less total volume and may minimize edema. Care should be taken to monitor hemodynamics with an understanding that central venous pressure reflects the outflow pressure for the liver and elevation may be associated with hepatic congestion. Serial measurements of hemoglobin are indicated to detect ongoing bleeding. Vasopressors may be used to restore arterial tone and ensure adequate perfusion pressure. However, cirrhosis is often associated with cardiomyopathy and left ventricular function will be compromised by excessive afterload. Norepinephrine offers balanced alpha and beta adrenergic support to preserve cardiac output and maintain mean arterial pressure (MAP). Vasopressin allows a lower norepinephrine infusion rate. Boluses of ephedrine or phenylephrine counter transient decreases in arterial tone caused by sedatives, narcotic analgesics, or volatile anesthetics. We target a MAP greater than 65 to 70 mm Hg unless a higher pressure is needed to perfuse a very congested liver allograft, evidenced by high resistive indices detected and monitored by Doppler ultrasonography postoperatively.

- Electrocardiogram: Evidence of ischemia and/or electrolyte disturbance should be assessed for by a post-LT electrocardiogram.
- Respiratory status: High minute ventilation may have been required intraoperatively to compensate for metabolic acidosis and the initial ICU mechanical ventilatory settings should take account of this, with adjustments as required based on ABGs. A lung-protective ventilatory strategy with tidal volume adjusted for ideal body weight is used intraoperatively and postoperatively. Patients are prone to atelectasis and positive end expiratory pressure (PEEP) is routinely utilized, titrated to minimize increases in right atrial pressure but sufficient to avoid atelectrauma. A chest radiograph should be taken to evaluate the lung parenchyma and pleural cavities and assess the position of the tracheal tube, vascular access devices, nasogastric tube, and chest tube if present.
- Neuromuscular blockade: Depending on the planned time to extubation, neostigmine (with glycopyrrolate) may be administered when appropriate to reverse the neuromuscular blockade. An adequate level of sedation should be ensured while pharmacologic paralysis is present.
- Initial postoperative analgesia is usually provided by fentanyl boluses or a low dose fentanyl infusion.
- Sedation, usually with propofol infusion, should be continued in the early postoperative period while the initial ICU assessment takes place and hemodynamic stability is ensured.
- Abdominal assessment: Abdominal examination and measurement of abdominal girth on ICU admission may be used for comparison later if intra-abdominal bleeding is suspected. The nature, volume, and rate of abdominal drain output will guide the need for transfusion, correction of coagulopathy, or return to the OR for bleeding. If a bile drainage tube is in situ, the presence of golden-brown bile is a sign of allograft function.
- Temperature management: Despite intraoperative warming techniques, the LT recipient often develops hypothermia because of redistribution and evaporative heat loss and the use of ice and cold organ preservation solution. Active warming to achieve normothermia should occur in the ICU.
- Urine output: Production of 0.5 mL/kg per hour in an adult is appropriate, although urine output greater than this is often seen and is usually a good sign. Initial oliguria should prompt consideration of volume administration and/or investigation for cardiac dysfunction. A significant number of patients may

have had pretransplant renal dysfunction (see later in this article) and urine output is one of a number of parameters used to assess the need for initiation, continuation, or cessation of dialysis. Diabetes insipidus is rare in the LT recipient unless the patient has succumbed to brain death in the peri-transplant period.

- Initial laboratory analyses: Early postoperative laboratory analyses (which are often drawn according to an institutional protocol) should include a complete blood count, electrolytes, blood urea nitrogen and creatinine, international normalized ratio, activated partial thromboplastin time, fibrinogen, and arterial blood gas analysis. A thromboelastogram (TEG) also may be useful.
- Discussion with surgeon and anesthesiologist: Information regarding intubation, anesthesia management, ease of vascular access, hemodynamic response to fluids or drugs, nature of the surgical dissection and anastomoses, organ ischemia time, and appearance and initial function of the allograft should be sought.
- Discussion with patient family: The surgical team will typically have discussed intraoperative events with the patient's family, but an initial brief communication with the ICU team will help establish rapport and lessen anxiety.

Protocols for Postoperative Care

Transplant programs have embraced the concepts of clinical pathways, "bundles," and protocols in an effort to increase adherence to best practice, and early postoperative management is suitable for use of such practices. Ventilator "bundles," ventilator weaning protocols, glycemic control pathways, electrolyte replacement order sets, and scheduled performance of laboratory and radiologic testing may be used in the postoperative care of the LT recipient.[15–17]

Graft Function

Satisfactory function of the new liver is associated with resolution of metabolic acidosis and coagulopathy, a decrease in bleeding, and stabilization of hemodynamics. Initially high serum transaminase concentrations (with aspartate aminotransferase peaking first within 24 hours) are due to reperfusion injury and should fall during the first postoperative week. A cholestatic phase ensues and a bilirubin peak by 7 to 10 days is associated with a rise in alkaline phosphatase, which can persist. Cholestasis associated with worsening coagulopathy and encephalopathy heralds graft failure. Bedside ultrasound with hepatic blood vessel Doppler examination is usually performed on the day of surgery or on the first postoperative day, and may be especially useful if the procedure has been technically difficult or if the allograft is functioning poorly to identify vascular abnormalities that might be amenable to treatment. "Initial poor function" is due to ischemic insults suffered during procurement, preservation, and implantation, and will usually resolve with appropriate physiologic support. The use of expanded criteria donors has increased the implantation of "marginal" allografts, which are more likely to be initially dysfunctional. "Primary nonfunction" is a rare, more serious immunologic insult that begins in the OR and causes failure of the liver graft, requiring emergent retransplantation.[18] Graft dysfunction causes lactic acidosis, acute kidney injury, hyperkalemia, hypoglycemia, encephalopathy, and increasing transaminase levels. Unfortunately, biochemical parameters alone often do not distinguish vascular impairment, biliary disruption, and rejection. Consequently, a low threshold should be maintained for evaluation with Doppler ultrasonography, cholangiography, and liver biopsy. Acute cellular rejection is much less common with the routine use of tacrolimus for immunosuppression. It is also less common in the elderly and the critically ill recipient.[19] A sudden reversal in falling bilirubin and an uptick in aminotransferases at 5 to 10 days after transplantation should prompt consideration of rejection.

SYSTEM-BASED CONSIDERATIONS FOR POSTOPERATIVE MANAGEMENT
Respiratory System Considerations

As detailed in Respiratory Complication in Liver Disease by Ramalingam VS, Ansari S and Fisher M, in this issue, there are many reasons for pretransplant hypoxemia in patients with liver disease, some of which may affect ICU management.

Weaning from mechanical ventilatory support after "routine" liver transplantation
In most patients, prolonged mechanical ventilatory support after LT is not necessary and patients can be weaned within a few hours of the end of surgery.[20] The timing of extubation after LT remains a subject of some controversy.[21,22] In a variety of surgical practices (eg, cardiac, thoracic) early extubation after major surgery has been demonstrated to be safe and to decrease costs. Application of such principles to LT is appropriate and careful intraoperative drug selection and drug dosing has allowed extubation of most patients within 8 hours of LT. Ventilator weaning protocols allow nurse and respiratory therapist engagement modifying sedation depth and ventilator settings to allow extubation following clinician order. Some clinicians have taken an even more aggressive approach to ventilator liberation. They argue that immediate postoperative extubation (IPE) in the OR or recovery room is safe and, by improving splanchnic and hepatic blood flow and reducing the risk of ventilator-associated pneumonia, is beneficial. IPE may allow the patient to avoid ICU admission, reducing hospital length of stay and ICU-associated costs.[20,23–25] However, safe avoidance of the ICU after LT requires careful redirection of nursing resources and very close collaboration among the anesthesiology, ICU, and ward teams. Indeed, others contend that a period of postoperative ventilation allows graft function to be consolidated with less sympathetic activation and protects the recipient from the risks of atelectasis, aspiration, or reintubation for surgical reexploration if required.[3,20,22] "Delayed" extubation (ie, non-IPE) allows for ensurance of hemodynamic stability and hemostasis and facilitates the titration of opiate analgesics for postoperative pain, without concern for hypoventilation or airway compromise in the early postoperative period. The availability of postanesthesia care unit (PACU) resources and a suitable non-ICU surgical ward are principal barriers to the implementation of IPE. Costs of PACU recovery versus ICU stay intersect at approximately 6 hours.[23] In a study involving 7 centers (5 in the United States, 2 in Europe), 391 patients were extubated within 1 hour of completion of LT surgery.[26] Adverse events within 72 hours occurred in 7.7% of them. The events were mostly minor and there was considerable intercenter variability. Early extubation is performed in 60% to 70% of LT cases in some centers, with avoidance of ICU admission in many of those cases, and reduction in costs.[23,24,27,28] To date, there has not been a randomized trial of immediate versus early versus delayed extubation after LT.

Respiratory compromise after liver transplantation
In many cases, patients are unsuitable for early extubation. Ongoing bleeding, significant acidosis, and large intraoperative transfusion requirements leading to volume overload or airway edema may compromise the ability to successfully wean. Patients may require diuresis for hypervolemia, drainage of pleural effusions, or administration of acetazolamide to offset hypoventilation secondary to metabolic alkalosis that develops after citrate metabolism.[29,30] Preoperative patient factors,

such as encephalopathy, the need for preoperative respiratory support, severe malnutrition, or sepsis, may also render a recipient ineligible for "fast tracking." Cirrhosis-related lung disease, such as hepatopulmonary syndrome (see later in this article) or alpha-one antitrypsin deficiency, coupled with the diaphragm dysfunction that occurs as a result of the surgical procedure, will also compromise weaning. Faenza and colleagues[31] identified the presence of early postoperative impairment of Pao_2/Fio_2 as a predictor of prolonged postoperative ventilation. Lung injury is common in patients with liver failure. It has also been recognized in patients who undergo complex abdominal surgeries unrelated to LT and recognized as a consequence of blood transfusion.[32,33] Therefore, LT recipients are at high risk for developing lung injury (see later in this article). Ventilation should be undertaken with an eye toward minimizing lung injury.

Ancillary strategies will support efforts at minimizing atelectasis and allowing early extubation. These include weaning sedation, early mobilization, and advancing physical and occupational therapy as tolerated. The strategies can be implemented even in the patient requiring vasopressor support. Evidence-based weaning strategies should be used in patients who are difficult to wean. Daily T-piece trials or pressure support weaning are more effective than intermittent mandatory ventilation weaning in these circumstances.[34] Although the benefits of tracheostomy are recognized, it is unusual for LT recipients to require tracheostomy and if performed, usually 2 to 3 weeks of ventilatory support are allowed to pass first. Percutaneous tracheostomy is gaining acceptance among the ICU community, and there is some experience in transplant recipients.[35,36]

Acute respiratory distress syndrome after liver transplantation

LT recipients may develop acute respiratory distress syndrome (ARDS) as a result of the surgical insult, reperfusion injury or graft dysfunction, transfusion-related acute lung injury, sepsis, aspiration (preoperative or less likely during induction of anesthesia), or treatment with monoclonal antibody therapy.[37,38] Pretransplant ARDS may disqualify a patient from receiving a transplant, except in the case of ALF-related ARDS.[39] The ARDSNet ARMA trial excluded patients with severe liver disease, although a lung-protective strategy with prescribed tidal volume based on ideal body weight strategy is appropriate in post-LT ARDS.[40] Although the optimal level is uncertain, PEEP is an established method to improve oxygenation in mechanically ventilated patients and is especially useful in patients with ARDS.[41,42] PEEP can be titrated to a level that exceeds pleural pressure. Pleural pressure can be estimated by measuring esophageal pressure.[43] Although there are concerns that the use of PEEP in a patient with a newly engrafted liver may increase hepatic engorgement and compromise function, hepatic inflow and outflow of the transplanted livers are not impaired by PEEP levels up to approximately 10 cm H_2O.[44–46] The effects of higher PEEP levels are uncertain. Preservation of the liver graft needs to be accompanied by survival of the patient, so if a higher PEEP level is required to sustain oxygenation, it should be applied. Furthermore, the reduced compliance of the ARDS-injured lungs may offset some transmission of pressure. There is minimal published experience with the use of permissive hypercapnia and high-frequency oscillation in patients after LT. Reports of the use of prone positioning provide conflicting messages.[47,48]

Perioperative hepatopulmonary syndrome

Hepatopulmonary syndrome (HPS) is discussed in detail in Respiratory Complication in Liver Disease by Ramalingam VS, Ansari S and Fisher M, in this issue. In the perioperative period, a failure of the Pao_2 to adequately increase with administration of

100% O_2 may result in critical hypoxemia.[49–51] Even in patients who respond satisfactorily, postoperative weaning from mechanical ventilation may be challenging and oxygen dependence may persist for weeks to months after extubation.[52,53] Severe HPS-related hypoxemia in the ICU may respond to Trendelenburg positioning or administration of intravenous methylene blue or inhaled N(G)-nitro-L-arginine methyl ester.[54,55]

Ventilator-associated pneumonia and noninvasive ventilation

Patients who spend a short period of time on the ventilator after "routine" LT are unlikely to develop ventilator-associated pneumonia (VAP). In those requiring longer perioperative periods of ventilation, the semi-recumbent position should be used assuming there are no hemodynamic contraindications.[56] If VAP is suspected, investigation should proceed along established guidelines, and include bronchoalveolar lavage with immunocompromised host protocol.[57] Although not routinely used in patients after LT, noninvasive ventilation may be initiated immediately after extubation in patients not thought to be ready for complete withdrawal of ventilatory support but in whom there is a desire to limit the duration of invasive mechanical ventilation.[58] In addition, the technique is useful in patients in whom there is a desire to avoid intubation or reintubation while a reversible problem (eg, volume overload) is treated.[59]

Cardiovascular System Considerations

The circulatory system implications of severe liver disease are detailed in The Circulatory System in Liver Disease by Hollenberg SM and Waldman B, in this issue. The hyperdynamic, vasodilated preoperative state persists into the early postoperative period and failure to see it may indicate volume depletion or myocardial dysfunction.[60] Despite the apparently vigorous myocardium, the heart may not tolerate large volumes of fluid. Pharmacologic augmentation of systemic blood pressure using norepinephrine and/or vasopressin or inotropic support by epinephrine, dobutamine, or dopamine may be required postoperatively to ensure adequate perfusion of the liver graft and other vital organs.

A small percentage of patients develop posttransplant cardiomyopathy, which usually presents a few days after transplantation with pulmonary edema–induced respiratory failure as a result of left ventricular dysfunction.[61] On occasion, apical ballooning suggests Takotsubo or stress-induced cardiomyopathy.[62,63] The condition is usually reversible and supportive treatment includes invasive or noninvasive respiratory support, inotropes, and diuretics. Rarely, cardiac tamponade develops after LT because of violation of the pericardium by the "Mercedes incision," inadvertent inclusion of the right atrium in the superior anastomosis to the inferior vena cava, or cardiac perforation by central venous cannula.

Elevated troponins seen postoperatively are most likely related to intraoperative demand ischemia rather than coronary artery thrombosis.[64] Acute coronary syndrome due to acute obstruction of a coronary artery is unusual. Discussion about percutaneous coronary intervention, antiplatelet therapy, and anticoagulation should include the cardiologist, intensivist, and LT surgeon.

Hypertension and arrhythmias

Post-LT hypertension may be due to fluid overload, pain, anxiety, preexisting chronic hypertension, or administration of cyclosporine and tacrolimus. Treatment is usually initiated when blood pressure is greater than 160/100 mm Hg. Rapidly acting agents with short duration of action (eg, labetalol, hydralazine) are preferred initially in the ICU with longer-acting enteral agents administered later after achievement of hemodynamic stability. Arrhythmias may occur secondary to hypercapnia, hypoxemia, electrolyte imbalances, metabolic acidosis, myocardial dysfunction, or irritation by central venous catheters. Atrial fibrillation may develop due to perioperative fluid shifts and electrolyte abnormalities.[65] Beta-blockers and calcium antagonists are preferred over amiodarone because of the drug's potential hepatotoxicity.

Portopulmonary hypertension

Patients with portopulmonary hypertension (PPH) are at increased risk perioperatively. Exacerbation of PPH with subsequent right ventricular dysfunction and congestion of the hepatic veins poses a risk to both graft and patient survival. It is imperative that preoperative treatments, such as sildenafil, bosentan, and intravenous epoprostenol, be continued perioperatively.[66–77] Weaning after transplantation can take weeks. As additional therapy, inhaled nitric oxide (at doses of up to 80 ppm) can be delivered into the breathing circuit intraoperatively and postoperatively to reduce pulmonary artery pressures. In extreme circumstances, placement of a right ventricular assist device or performance of an atrial septostomy have been described.[74,78,79]

The Nervous System

Assuming the patient is extubated quickly, propofol and fentanyl infusions are discontinued and analgesia provided with a patient-controlled analgesia device administering fentanyl or a longer-acting opiate such as hydromorphone. Transition to enteral analgesics using opiates such as oxycodone or nonopiates can usually occur within 1 to 2 days. Although LT recipients may have significant pain, their analgesic requirements are often less than the analgesic requirements for other upper abdominal procedures.[80] If sedation requirements are prolonged (eg, ARDS after transplantation) propofol or dexmedetomidine may be used. Infusions of benzodiazepines should be avoided if possible, especially in patients with marginal graft function, in whom their metabolism may be delayed.

Neurologic dysfunction occurs in as many as 25% of LT recipients in the perioperative period.[81–84] The most common problems are encephalopathy and seizures. In patients with an intact sensorium, the speed of awakening is related to redistribution and metabolism of anesthetic and sedative agents. Those who had preoperative encephalopathy have delayed awakening, the duration being proportional to the severity and duration of preexisting encephalopathy. Postoperative delirium is associated with worse outcomes in LT recipients.[85]

Management of cerebral edema in ALF is by conventional means and includes minimization of noxious stimuli, avoidance of mechanical obstruction to cerebral venous outflow, administration of sedative agents, such as propofol, mild hyperventilation, mannitol or hypertonic saline administration, use of the reverse Trendelenburg position, and potentially, moderate hypothermia.[86–93] If initiated preoperatively, such therapies may need to be continued into the postoperative period, until a functional liver allograft leads to a reduction in intracranial pressure (ICP). There are rare reports, however, of cerebral herniation intraoperatively and in the early postoperative period, which is a devastating complication as it will result in the death of the recipient and loss of an organ that could have been used for another patient. In patients transplanted for ALF, cautious weaning of sedation should occur postoperatively, guided by an ICP monitor if there is one in situ.

Central pontine myelinolysis (CPM), a devastating condition associated with rapid alterations of serum sodium and osmolality is less frequent today because of awareness of the condition, less frequent administration of sodium bicarbonate, and use of nonsodium buffers such as tromethamine.[82,94–97] Postoperative seizures are unusual but may be related to intracranial infection or hemorrhage, severe hyponatremia or hypocalcemia, or calcineurin inhibitors.

Renal Considerations

Renal impairment is commonly seen in patients with liver disease and may occur before or after LT. In some cases, a combined liver-kidney transplantation is performed. Hepatorenal syndrome (HRS) is only one of a number of causes of renal dysfunction.[98] It generally recovers after LT unless irreversible renal damage has occurred. Other causes seen perioperatively include pre–renal azotemia due to hypovolemia, hypotension, and cardiac dysfunction, or acute tubular necrosis due to sepsis, or an inflammatory state caused by the surgical procedure.[99] Administration of large volumes of chloride-containing fluids also may be associated with renal damage.[100] Kidney biopsy will identify patients with structural damage, the absence of which correlates with recovery after liver-alone transplantation.[101] The procedure is associated with morbidity, which limits its widespread application.

Hyperkalemia may develop acutely intraoperatively around the time of reperfusion and may also occur perioperatively with transfusion of large volumes of packed red blood cells. In patients with marginal renal function, washing of the red cells to remove potassium should be performed before transfusion. Treatment of hyperkalemia is by conventional methods including administration of calcium, insulin/dextrose, sodium bicarbonate, beta-2 agonists, and furosemide in addition to consideration of treatment with sodium polystyrene sulfonate or dialysis.

New-onset postoperative renal dysfunction may also indicate severe graft dysfunction or primary nonfunction. More than 30% of patients with preoperative renal failure require hemodialysis in the short term, and approximately 5% need chronic therapy. Continuous renal replacement therapy is the method of choice in hemodynamically unstable patients, and has theoretic advantages in patients with elevated ICP or PPH. It may be continued in the OR during the operative period allowing intraoperative fluid removal and reduction of liver engorgement when a patient is anuric, and an improved ability to prevent and treat hyperkalemia and metabolic acidosis.[102,103]

Metabolic Considerations

Perioperative hyperglycemia is caused by surgical stress, the insulin resistance associated with liver failure, and administration of steroids and exogenous catecholamines. Control of hyperglycemia in the perioperative period and in critically ill patients has been a subject of considerable debate over the past decade.[104–107] There are insufficient data regarding peritransplant glycemic control, although it has been suggested that graft function may be affected by plasma glucose levels.[108–113] Perioperative hypoglycemia is of great concern because of the predisposition to its development in patients with liver dysfunction and altered glycogen stores, and especially those with ALF. Continuous infusion is typically initiated in the OR to maintain glycemic control and continued postoperatively. When used in conjunction with hourly glucose checks, this practice appears safe.[114] Hypoglycemia, if it occurs, should be treated with boluses of 50% dextrose, continuous infusions of 5% or 10% dextrose, and adjustment of the insulin algorithms that may be in use.

More than half of patients awaiting LT have moderate to severe protein calorie malnutrition and this is likely to worsen perioperatively.[115,116] Brisk return of gastrointestinal function usually occurs, so re-initiation of oral intake can usually occur within the first couple of days after surgery. Some surgeons initiate nasogastric or nasojejunal feeding in the immediate posttransplant period to preserve gut mucosal integrity. The use of total parenteral nutrition is usually unnecessary and is less desirable.

Perioperative hypocalcemia may occur due to chelation of calcium by the citrate preservative in packed red blood cells. In recipients of living donor and split liver grafts, phosphate repletion will be required for the regeneration of liver parenchyma.[117] Although relative adrenal insufficiency is possible in patients with severe liver disease, the large intraoperative dose of steroids usually administered in the OR will provide adequate exogenous glucocorticoid levels, even if endogenous levels are insufficient.

Coagulation Management

Coagulopathy results from inadequate clotting factor synthesis, hypersplenism, and fibrinolysis, as well as hypocalcemia and dilution. Perioperatively, the risk of bleeding must be balanced against the risk of hepatic artery or portal vein thrombosis. A functioning liver allograft will soon start to normalize coagulation parameters, but blood products, including coagulation factors, may be required to stop intraoperative and postoperative bleeding. Thrombocytopenia is seen in virtually all recipients after transplantation, with lowest levels seen on the third and fourth postoperative days. A scheme for perioperative coagulation management is provided in **Fig. 1**.

Immunosuppression

Immunosuppression is started in the OR. The specific regimen varies by institution, but a typical regimen includes corticosteroids, mycophenolate mofetil, and a calcineurin inhibitor, either tacrolimus or cyclosporine. It is essential in the perioperative

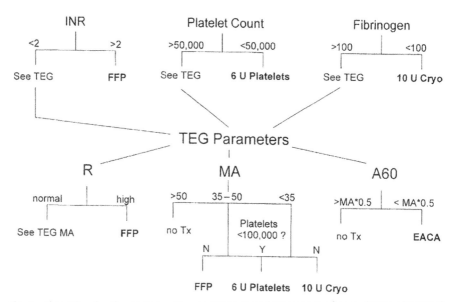

Fig. 1. Algorithm for the perioperative assessment and treatment of coagulation abnormalities in patients undergoing orthotopic liver transplantation. A60, TEG amplitude 60 minutes after the time of MA; Cryo, cryoprecipitate; EACA, ε-aminocaproic acid; FFP, fresh frozen plasma; MA, TEG maximal amplitude; R, TEG reaction time; TEG, thromboelastogram; Tx, treatment. (*From* Stapelfeldt W. Liver, kidney, pancreas transplantation. In: Murray MJ, Coursin DB, Pearl RG, et al, editors. Critical care medicine: perioperative management. 2nd edition. Philadelphia: Lippincott Williams and Wilkins; 2002. p. 728.)

period when multiple teams may be involved to specifically determine where responsibility for immunosuppressant ordering and administration lies. An ICU or transplant pharmacist is a valuable addition to the team of care providers. Rejection, unless it is primary nonfunction, is usually not seen during the first week after transplantation and so is not usually an ICU issue.[118–120] Rejection is also uncommon in the elderly.[19,121]

Infectious Disease Issues

LT candidates may have become weakened and colonized with resistant organisms and subsequently receive immunosuppressants, so it is not surprising that infection is the leading cause of death after LT. Infection is not, however, the most common cause in the postoperative period. Prophylactic antibiotics (usually a third-generation cephalosporin) are administered intraoperatively to decrease the risk of surgical site infections. Most posttransplant infections affect either the lungs or the abdominal cavity. Early respiratory infections may be caused by gram-negative enteric organisms or fungi such as *Candida* species or even *Aspergillus*.[122]

POSTOPERATIVE COMPLICATIONS
Postoperative Hemorrhage

Within the first 24 to 48 hours after LT, approximately 10% of patients require reoperation because of ongoing bleeding.[123–125] Signs include tachycardia, hypotension, abdominal distension, oliguria, elevated bladder and airway pressures, brisk drain output (unless clotted), and failure of the hematocrit to rise appropriately after transfusion. If brisk bleeding is ongoing, aggressive correction of coagulation abnormalities is usually necessary to decrease "medical" bleeding. Discussion between the critical care and surgical teams is important to ensure expeditious transfer back to the OR if required. At laparotomy, identifiable sources of bleeding include vascular anastomoses, the cystic bed, and liver lacerations, among others. Most commonly, however, a major bleeding site is not identified, the abdomen is simply washed out, and the patient returned to the ICU. Recipients of living donor LTs or split liver grafts are at greater risk of bleeding because of the presence of large, raw surfaces. Endovascular intervention to control bleeding has been described but is not typical.[126,127]

Vascular, Biliary, and Wound Complications

Complications related to vascular anastomoses occur in 6% to 12% of recipients.[127] Thrombosis is the most common problem, although pseudoaneurysm, stenosis, and dissection may occur. A balance must be maintained between optimization of coagulation parameters to control bleeding and the danger of thrombus formation, especially in the hepatic artery and portal vein. Postoperative hepatic artery thrombosis may cause a rapid clinical deterioration with markedly elevated transaminases. More indolent presentations can also occur, including ischemia of the common bile duct. The development of hepatic necrosis requires retransplantation. Prophylactic prostaglandin E1 ("alprostadil") may be used to preserve patency if there is concern about the nature of the hepatic artery anastomosis.[128] Clinical presentation of the (less common) portal vein thrombosis includes ascites, variceal bleeding, and severe liver dysfunction. If thrombosis of a vascular anastomosis occurs, prompt return to the OR for surgical intervention may salvage the graft. Biliary complications occur in 6% to 34% of patients and the incidence is higher in recipients of partial LTs. Postoperative bile leaks may present with fever, abdominal pain, and peritonitis and often require surgical repair. Obstruction is usually a later complication, not seen in the ICU. Wound infections and dehiscences, if they occur, usually do so after day 5 and are not typically ICU issues.

Readmission to the Intensive Care Unit

"Routine" LT recipients are usually ready for dismissal from the ICU within 24 hours of their procedure (and as discussed previously may not have been admitted to the ICU in the first place). Large-bore central and peripheral venous catheters are left in place in the early postoperative period but they are usually not required once a patient is suitable for transfer out of the ICU. Readmission to ICU is required in up to 20% of recipients, usually resulting from cardiopulmonary deterioration, although neurologic issues also may be responsible.[129,130] Hypervolemia, decreased inspiratory capacity, and increased respiratory rate at ICU discharge as well as a prolonged ICU course are associated with the need for readmission.[131] Readmission is associated with increased morbidity, costs, and graft failure.

SPECIAL CONSIDERATIONS

Postoperative ICU care of the recipient of living donor LT is similar to that of cadaveric donor transplants, although there may be more risk of bleeding from the large raw liver surface and of biliary complications. The arterial anastomosis is relatively small in such patients and may lead to a higher incidence of thrombosis. Congestion of the allograft due to portal venous hypertension or hepatic venous anastomotic problems or inadequate preservation of intrahepatic venous collaterals may occur and may cause liver dysfunction.[132,133] In many programs, donors spend the first night after their extended right hepatectomy in the ICU for careful postoperative monitoring.

SUMMARY

Advances in LT reflect the contributions of multiple specialties. The organ shortage and emphasis on long-term survival for the population of patients with liver disease have intensified the acuity of illness among recipients of LTs. Commonly, candidates for LT require intensive care for multiple organ dysfunction syndrome. Careful candidate selection requires close communication among the intensivist, hepatologist, LT surgeon, and LT anesthesiologist. Postoperative care requires similar communication about the status of the donated organ as well as the intraoperative course. Continued close communication among the transplant team members is essential.

REFERENCES

1. Findlay JY, Fix OK, Paugam-Burtz C, et al. Critical care of the end-stage liver disease patient awaiting liver transplantation. Liver Transpl 2011;17:496–510.
2. Knaak J, McVey M, Bazerbachi F, et al. Liver transplantation in patients with end-stage liver disease requiring intensive care unit admission and intubation. Liver Transpl 2015;21:761–7.
3. Xia VW, Taniguchi M, Steadman RH. The changing face of patients presenting for liver transplantation. Curr Opin Organ Transplant 2008;13:280–4.
4. Schumann R, Mandell MS, Mercaldo N, et al. Anesthesia for liver transplantation in United States academic centers: intraoperative practice. J Clin Anesth 2013; 25:542–50.
5. Liu LL, Niemann CU. Intraoperative management of liver transplant patients. Transplant Rev (Orlando) 2011;25:124–9.

6. Hannaman MJ, Hevesi ZG. Anesthesia care for liver transplantation. Transplant Rev (Orlando) 2011;25:36–43.

7. Hall TH, Dhir A. Anesthesia for liver transplantation. Semin Cardiothorac Vasc Anesth 2013;17:180–94.

8. Findlay JY, Jankowski CJ, Vasdev GM, et al. Fast track anesthesia for liver transplantation reduces postoperative ventilation time but not intensive care unit stay. Liver Transpl 2002;8:670–5.

9. Bernal W, Wendon J. Acute liver failure. N Engl J Med 2013;369:2525–34.

10. Lee WM, Stravitz RT, Larson AM. Introduction to the revised American Association for the Study of Liver Diseases position paper on acute liver failure 2011. Hepatology 2012;55:965–7.

11. Stravitz RT, Kramer AH, Davern T, et al. Intensive care of patients with acute liver failure: recommendations of the U.S. Acute Liver Failure Study Group. Crit Care Med 2007;35:2498–508.

12. Bernal W, Lee W, Wendon J, et al. Acute liver failure: a curable disease by 2024? J Hepatol 2015;62:S112–20.

13. Findlay JY, Long TR, Joyner MJ, et al. Changes in transfusion practice over time in adult patients undergoing liver transplantation. J Cardiothorac Vasc Anesth 2013;27:41–5.

14. Ramsay M. Justification for routine intensive care after liver transplantation. Liver Transpl 2013;19(Suppl 2):S1–5.

15. Ely EW, Bennett PA, Bowton DL, et al. Large scale implementation of a respiratory therapist-driven protocol for ventilator weaning. Am J Respir Crit Care Med 1999;159:439–46.

16. Todd SR, Sucher JF, Moore LJ, et al. A multidisciplinary protocol improves electrolyte replacement and its effectiveness. Am J Surg 2009;198:911–5.

17. Toledo AH, Carroll T, Arnold E, et al. Reducing liver transplant length of stay: a Lean Six Sigma approach. Prog Transplant 2013;23:350–64.

18. Brokelman W, Stel AL, Ploeg RJ. Risk factors for primary dysfunction after liver transplantation in the University of Wisconsin solution era. Transplant Proc 1999; 31:2087–90.

19. Aduen JF, Sujay B, Dickson RC, et al. Outcomes after liver transplant in patients aged 70 years or older compared with those younger than 60 years. Mayo Clin Proc 2009;84:973–8.

20. Ozier Y, Klinck JR. Anesthetic management of hepatic transplantation. Curr Opin Anaesthesiol 2008;21:391–400.

21. Mandell MS, Campsen J, Zimmerman M, et al. The clinical value of early extubation. Curr Opin Organ Transplant 2009;14:297–302.

22. Steadman RH. Con: immediate extubation for liver transplantation. J Cardiothorac Vasc Anesth 2007;21:756–7.

23. Taner CB, Willingham DL, Bulatao IG, et al. Is a mandatory intensive care unit stay needed after liver transplantation? Feasibility of fast-tracking to the surgical ward after liver transplantation. Liver Transpl 2012;18:361–9.

24. Mandell MS, Lezotte D, Kam I, et al. Reduced use of intensive care after liver transplantation: patient attributes that determine early transfer to surgical wards. Liver Transpl 2002;8:682–7.

25. Aniskevich S, Pai SL. Fast track anesthesia for liver transplantation: review of the current practice. World J Hepatol 2015;7:2303–8.

26. Mandell MS, Stoner TJ, Barnett R, et al. A multicenter evaluation of safety of early extubation in liver transplant recipients. Liver Transpl 2007;13:1557–63.

27. Biancofiore G, Romanelli AM, Bindi ML, et al. Very early tracheal extubation without predetermined criteria in a liver transplant recipient population. Liver Transpl 2001;7:777–82.

28. Glanemann M, Langrehr J, Kaisers U, et al. Postoperative tracheal extubation after orthotopic liver transplantation. Acta Anaesthesiol Scand 2001;45:333–9.

29. Carton EG, Plevak DJ, Kranner PW, et al. Perioperative care of the liver transplant patient: part 1. Anesth Analg 1994;78:120–33.

30. Carton EG, Plevak DJ, Kranner PW, et al. Perioperative care of the liver transplant patient: part 2. Anesth Analg 1994;78:382–99.

31. Faenza S, Ravaglia MS, Cimatti M, et al. Analysis of the causal factors of prolonged mechanical ventilation after orthotopic liver transplant. Transplant Proc 2006;38:1131–4.

32. Looney MR, Roubinian N, Gajic O, et al. Prospective study on the clinical course and outcomes in transfusion-related acute lung injury. Crit Care Med 2014;42:1676–87.

33. Manez R, Kusne S, Martin M, et al. The impact of blood transfusion on the occurrence of pneumonitis in primary cytomegalovirus infection after liver transplantation. Transfusion 1993;33:594–7.

34. Frustos-Vivar F, Esteban A, Paezteguia C, et al. Outcome of mechanically ventilated patients who require a tracheostomy. Crit Care Med 2005;33:290–8.

35. Pirat A, Zeyneloglu P, Candan S, et al. Percutaneous dilational tracheotomy in solid-organ transplant recipients. Transplant Proc 2004;36:221–3.

36. Waller EA, Aduen JF, Kramer DJ, et al. Safety of percutaneous dilatational tracheostomy with direct bronchoscopic guidance for solid organ allograft recipients. Mayo Clin Proc 2007;82:1502–8.

37. Yost CS, Matthay MA, Gropper MA. Etiology of acute pulmonary edema during liver transplantation: a series of cases with analysis of the edema fluid. Chest 2001;119:219–23.

38. Sachdeva A, Matuschak GM. Diffuse alveolar hemorrhage following alemtuzumab. Chest 2008;133:1476–8.

39. Doyle HR, Marino IR, Miro A, et al. Adult respiratory distress syndrome secondary to end-stage liver disease—successful outcome following liver transplantation. Transplantation 1993;55:292–6.

40. Ventilation with lower tidal volumes as compared with traditional tidal volumes for acute lung injury and the acute respiratory distress syndrome. The acute respiratory distress syndrome network. N Engl J Med 2000;342:1301–8.

41. Brower RG, Lanken PN, MacIntyre N, et al. Higher versus lower positive endexpiratory pressures in patients with the acute respiratory distress syndrome. N Engl J Med 2004;351:327–36.

42. Villar J, Kacmarek R, Perez-Mendez L, et al. A high positive-end expiratory pressure, low tidal volume ventilatory strategy improves outcome in persistent acute respiratory distress syndrome: a randomized control trial. Crit Care Med 2006;34:1311–8.

43. Talmor D, Sarge T, Malhotra A, et al. Mechanical ventilation guided by esophageal pressure in acute lung injury. N Engl J Med 2008;359:2095–104.

44. Saner FH, Pavlakovic G, Gu Y, et al. Effects of positive end-expiratory pressure on systemic haemodynamics, with special interest to central venous and common iliac venous pressure in liver transplanted patients. Eur J Anaesthesiol 2006;23:766–71.

45. Saner FH, Olde Damink SW, Pavlakovic G, et al. Positive end-expiratory pressure induces liver congestion in living donor liver transplant patients: myth or fact. Transplantation 2008;85:1863–6.

46. Saner FH, Pavlakovic G, Gu Y, et al. Does PEEP impair the hepatic outflow in patients following liver transplantation? Intensive Care Med 2006;32:1584–90.

47. Sykes E, Cosgrove JF, Nesbitt ID, et al. Early noncardiogenic pulmonary edema and the use of PEEP and prone ventilation after emergency liver transplantation. Liver Transpl 2007;13:459–62.

48. De Schryver N, Castanares-Zapatero D, Laterre PF, et al. Prone positioning induced hepatic necrosis after liver transplantation. Intensive Care Med 2015; 41(10):1833.

49. Koch DG, Fallon MB. Hepatopulmonary syndrome. Clin Liver Dis 2014;18: 407–20.

50. Fauconnet P, Klopfenstein CE, Schiffer E. Hepatopulmonary syndrome: the anaesthetic considerations. Eur J Anaesthesiol 2013;30:721–30.

51. Hoeper MM, Krowka MJ, Strassburg CP. Portopulmonary hypertension and hepatopulmonary syndrome. Lancet 2004;363:1461–8.

52. Collisson EA, Nourmand H, Fraiman MH, et al. Retrospective analysis of the results of liver transplantation for adults with severe hepatopulmonary syndrome. Liver Transpl 2002;8:925–31.

53. Taille C, Cadranel J, Bellocq A, et al. Liver transplantation for hepatopulmonary syndrome: a ten-year experience in Paris, France. Transplantation 2003;75: 1482–9.

54. Schenk P, Madl C, Rezaie-Majd S, et al. Methylene blue improves the hepatopulmonary syndrome. Ann Intern Med 2000;133:701–6.

55. Brussino L, Bucca C, Morello M, et al. Effect on dyspnoea and hypoxaemia of inhaled N(G)-nitro-L-arginine methyl ester in hepatopulmonary syndrome. Lancet 2003;362:43–4.

56. Dodek P, Keenan S, Cook D, et al. Evidence-based clinical practice guideline for the prevention of ventilator-associated pneumonia. Ann Intern Med 2004; 141:305–13.

57. Chastre J, Fagon JY. Ventilator-associated pneumonia. Am J Respir Crit Care Med 2002;165:867–903.

58. Ferrer M. Non-invasive ventilation as a weaning tool. Minerva Anestesiol 2005; 71:243–7.

59. Antonelli M, Conti G, Bufi M, et al. Noninvasive ventilation for treatment of acute respiratory failure in patients undergoing solid organ transplantation: a randomized trial. JAMA 2000;283:235–41.

60. Nasraway SA, Klein RD, Spanier TB, et al. Hemodynamic correlates of outcome in patients undergoing orthotopic liver transplantation. Evidence for early postoperative myocardial depression. Chest 1995;107:218–24.

61. Sampathkumar P, Lerman A, Kim BY, et al. Post-liver transplantation myocardial dysfunction. Liver Transpl Surg 1998;4:399–403.

62. Adar T, Chen S, Mizrahi M. A heartbreaking case of Wilson's disease: Takotsubo cardiomyopathy complicating fulminant hepatic failure. Transpl Int 2014;27: e109–11.

63. Harika R, Bermas K, Hughes C, et al. Cardiac arrest after liver transplantation in a patient with Takotsubo cardiomyopathy. Br J Anaesth 2014;112:594–5.

64. Findlay JY, Keegan MT, Pellikka PP, et al. Preoperative dobutamine stress echocardiography, intraoperative events, and intraoperative myocardial injury in liver transplantation. Transplant Proc 2005;37:2209–13.

65. Xia VW, Worapot A, Huang S, et al. Postoperative atrial fibrillation in liver transplantation. Am J Transplant 2015;15:687–94.
66. Cartin-Ceba R, Krowka MJ. Portopulmonary hypertension. Clin Liver Dis 2014; 18:421–38.
67. Ghofrani HA, Rose F, Schermuly RT, et al. Oral sildenafil as long-term adjunct therapy to inhaled iloprost in severe pulmonary arterial hypertension. J Am Coll Cardiol 2003;42:158–64.
68. Channick RN, Simonneau G, Sitbon O, et al. Effects of the dual endothelin-receptor antagonist bosentan in patients with pulmonary hypertension: a randomised placebo-controlled study. Lancet 2001;358:1119–23.
69. Kuo PC, Johnson LB, Plotkin JS, et al. Continuous intravenous infusion of epoprostenol for the treatment of portopulmonary hypertension. Transplantation 1997;63:604–6.
70. Kaddis JS, Olack BJ, Sowinski J, et al. Human pancreatic islets and diabetes research. JAMA 2009;301:1580–7.
71. Kim BJ, Lee SC, Park SW, et al. Characteristics and prevalence of intrapulmonary shunt detected by contrast echocardiography with harmonic imaging in liver transplant candidates. Am J Cardiol 2004;94:525–8.
72. Kim WR, Krowka MJ, Plevak DJ, et al. Accuracy of Doppler echocardiography in the assessment of pulmonary hypertension in liver transplant candidates. Liver Transpl 2000;6:453–8.
73. Krowka MJ, Mandell MS, Ramsay MA, et al. Hepatopulmonary syndrome and portopulmonary hypertension: a report of the multicenter liver transplant database. Liver Transpl 2004;10:174–82.
74. Krowka MJ, Plevak DJ, Findlay JY, et al. Pulmonary hemodynamics and perioperative cardiopulmonary-related mortality in patients with portopulmonary hypertension undergoing liver transplantation. Liver Transpl 2000;6:443–50.
75. Hoeper MM, Gall H, Seyfarth HJ, et al. Long-term outcome with intravenous iloprost in pulmonary arterial hypertension. Eur Respir J 2009;34:132–7.
76. Sussman N, Kaza V, Barshes N, et al. Successful liver transplantation following medical management of portopulmonary hypertension: a single-center series. Am J Transplant 2006;6:2177–82.
77. Ashfaq M, Chinnakotla S, Rogers L, et al. The impact of treatment of portopulmonary hypertension on survival following liver transplantation. Am J Transplant 2007;7:1258–64.
78. Findlay JY, Harrison BA, Plevak DJ, et al. Inhaled nitric oxide reduces pulmonary artery pressures in portopulmonary hypertension. Liver Transpl Surg 1999;5:381–7.
79. Ramsay MA, Spikes C, East CA, et al. The perioperative management of portopulmonary hypertension with nitric oxide and epoprostenol. Anesthesiology 1999;90:299–301.
80. Eisenach JC, Plevak DJ, Van Dyke RA, et al. Comparison of analgesic requirements after liver transplantation and cholecystectomy. Mayo Clin Proc 1989;64: 356–9.
81. Saner F, Gu Y, Minouchehr S, et al. Neurological complications after cadaveric and living donor liver transplantation. J Neurol 2006;253:612–7.
82. Ardizzone G, Arrigo A, Schellino M, et al. Neurological complications of liver cirrhosis and orthotopic liver transplant. Transplant Proc 2006;38:789–92.
83. Wijdicks EF. Impaired consciousness after liver transplantation. Liver Transpl Surg 1995;1:329–34.
84. Zivkovic SA. Neurologic complications after liver transplantation. World J Hepatol 2013;5:409–16.

85. Lescot T, Karvellas CJ, Chaudhury P, et al. Postoperative delirium in the intensive care unit predicts worse outcomes in liver transplant recipients. Can J Gastroenterol 2013;27:207–12.
86. Wijdicks EF, Nyberg SL. Propofol to control intracranial pressure in fulminant hepatic failure. Transplant Proc 2002;34:1220–2.
87. Wijdicks EF, Plevak DJ, Rakela J, et al. Clinical and radiologic features of cerebral edema in fulminant hepatic failure. Mayo Clin Proc 1995;70:119–24.
88. Wijdicks EF. The diagnosis of brain death. N Engl J Med 2001;344:1215–21.
89. Dmello D, Cruz-Flores S, Matuschak GM. Moderate hypothermia with intracranial pressure monitoring as a therapeutic paradigm for the management of acute liver failure: a systematic review. Intensive Care Med 2010;36:210–3.
90. Stravitz RT, Larsen FS. Therapeutic hypothermia for acute liver failure. Crit Care Med 2009;37:S258–64.
91. Daas M, Plevak DJ, Wijdicks EF, et al. Acute liver failure: results of a 5-year clinical protocol. Liver Transpl Surg 1995;1:210–9.
92. Jalan R, O Damink SW, Deutz NE, et al. Moderate hypothermia for uncontrolled intracranial hypertension in acute liver failure. Lancet 1999;354:1164–8.
93. Jalan R, Olde Damink SW, Deutz NE, et al. Moderate hypothermia prevents cerebral hyperemia and increase in intracranial pressure in patients undergoing liver transplantation for acute liver failure. Transplantation 2003;75:2034–9.
94. Lee EM, Kang JK, Yun SC, et al. Risk factors for central pontine and extrapontine myelinolysis following orthotopic liver transplantation. Eur Neurol 2009;62: 362–8.
95. Wijdicks EF, Blue PR, Steers JL, et al. Central pontine myelinolysis with stupor alone after orthotopic liver transplantation. Liver Transpl Surg 1996;2:14–6.
96. Bronster DJ, Emre S, Boccagni P, et al. Central nervous system complications in liver transplant recipients–incidence, timing, and long-term follow-up. Clin Transpl 2000;14:1–7.
97. Hudcova J, Ruthazer R, Bonney I, et al. Sodium homeostasis during liver transplantation and correlation with outcomes. Anesth Analg 2014;119:1420–8.
98. Gines P, Guevara M, Arroyo V, et al. Hepatorenal syndrome. Lancet 2003;362: 1819–27.
99. Cabezuelo JB, Ramirez P, Rios A, et al. Risk factors of acute renal failure after liver transplantation. Kidney Int 2006;69:1073–80.
100. Nadeem A, Salahuddin N, El Hazmi A, et al. Chloride-liberal fluids are associated with acute kidney injury after liver transplantation. Crit Care 2014;18:625.
101. Wadei HM, Geiger XJ, Cortese C, et al. Kidney allocation to liver transplant candidates with renal failure of undetermined etiology: role of percutaneous renal biopsy. Am J Transplant 2008;8:2618–26.
102. Gali B, Keegan M, Leung N, et al. Continuous renal replacement therapy during high risk liver transplantation. Liver Transpl 2006;12:C-117.
103. Townsend DR, Bagshaw SM, Jacka MJ, et al. Intraoperative renal support during liver transplantation. Liver Transpl 2009;15:73–8.
104. Akhtar S, Barash PG, Inzucchi SE. Scientific principles and clinical implications of perioperative glucose regulation and control. Anesth Analg 2010;110:478–97.
105. Finfer S, Chittock DR, Su SY, et al. Intensive versus conventional glucose control in critically ill patients. N Engl J Med 2009;360:1283–97.
106. Griesdale DE, de Souza RJ, van Dam RM, et al. Intensive insulin therapy and mortality among critically ill patients: a meta-analysis including NICE-SUGAR study data. CMAJ 2009;180:821–7.

107. Moghissi E, Korytkowski M, DiNardo M, et al. American Association of Clinical Endocrinologists and American Diabetes Association consensus statement on inpatient glycemic control. Endocr Pract 2009;15:353–69.

108. Marvin M, Morton V. Glycemic control and organ transplantation. J Diabetes Sci Technol 2009;3:1365–72.

109. Ammori JB, Sigakis M, Englesbe MJ, et al. Effect of intraoperative hyperglycemia during liver transplantation. J Surg Res 2007;140:227–33.

110. DeWolf AM, Kang YG, Todo S, et al. Glucose metabolism during liver transplantation in dogs. Anesth Analg 1987;66:76–80.

111. Atchison SR, Rettke SR, Fromme GA, et al. Plasma glucose concentrations during liver transplantation. Mayo Clin Proc 1989;64:241–5.

112. Hsaiky L, Bajjoka I, Patel D, et al. Postoperative use of intense insulin therapy in liver transplant recipients. Am J Transplant 2008;8(S2):260.

113. Marvin M, Rocca J, Farrington E, et al. Intensive perioperative insulin therapy in liver transplant patients—effective implementation with a computer-based dosage calculator. Am J Transplant 2006;6(S2):986.

114. Keegan MT, Vrchota JM, Haala PM, et al. Safety and effectiveness of intensive insulin protocol use in post-operative liver transplant recipients. Transplant Proc 2010;42:2617–24.

115. Stephenson GR, Moretti EW, El-Moalem H, et al. Malnutrition in liver transplant patients: preoperative subjective global assessment is predictive of outcome after liver transplantation. Transplantation 2001;72:666–70.

116. Nompleggi DJ, Bonkovsky HL. Nutritional supplementation in chronic liver disease: an analytical review. Hepatology 1994;19:518–33.

117. Pomposelli JJ, Pomfret EA, Burns DL, et al. Life-threatening hypophosphatemia after right hepatic lobectomy for live donor adult liver transplantation. Liver Transpl 2001;7:637–42.

118. Cohen SM. Current immunosuppression in liver transplantation. Am J Ther 2002; 9:119–25.

119. Buckley RH. Transplantation immunology: organ and bone marrow. J Allergy Clin Immunol 2003;111:S733–44.

120. Textor SC, Taler SJ, Canzanello VJ, et al. Posttransplantation hypertension related to calcineurin inhibitors. Liver Transpl 2000;6:521–30.

121. Manez R, Kusne S, Linden P, et al. Temporary withdrawal of immunosuppression for life-threatening infections after liver transplantation. Transplantation 1994;57: 149–51.

122. Aduen JF, Hellinger WC, Kramer DJ, et al. Spectrum of pneumonia in the current era of liver transplantation and its effect on survival. Mayo Clin Proc 2005;80: 1303–6.

123. Plevak DJ, Southorn PA, Narr BJ, et al. Intensive-care unit experience in the Mayo liver transplantation program: the first 100 cases. Mayo Clin Proc 1989; 64:433–45.

124. Liang TB, Bai XL, Li DL, et al. Early postoperative hemorrhage requiring urgent surgical reintervention after orthotopic liver transplantation. Transplant Proc 2007;39:1549–53.

125. Biancofiore G, Bindi ML, Romanelli AM, et al. Intra-abdominal pressure monitoring in liver transplant recipients: a prospective study. Intensive Care Med 2003;29:30–6.

126. Harman A, Boyvat F, Hasdogan B, et al. Endovascular treatment of active bleeding after liver transplant. Exp Clin Transplant 2007;5:596–600.

127. Cavallari A, Vivarelli M, Bellusci R, et al. Treatment of vascular complications following liver transplantation: multidisciplinary approach. Hepatogastroenterology 2001;48:179–83.
128. Gatta A, Dante A, Del Gaudio M, et al. The use of prostaglandins in the immediate postsurgical liver transplant period. Transplant Proc 2006;38:1092–5.
129. Levy MF, Greene L, Ramsay MA, et al. Readmission to the intensive care unit after liver transplantation. Crit Care Med 2001;29:18–24.
130. Kramer DJ. Intensive care unit frequent fliers: morbidity and cost. Crit Care Med 2001;29:207–8.
131. Cardoso FS, Karvellas CJ, Kneteman NM, et al. Respiratory rate at intensive care unit discharge after liver transplant is an independent risk factor for intensive care unit readmission within the same hospital stay: a nested case-control study. J Crit Care 2014;29:791–6.
132. Liu LU, Schiano TD. Adult live donor liver transplantation. Clin Liver Dis 2005;9: 767–86.
133. Trotter JF, Wachs M, Everson GT, et al. Adult-to-adult transplantation of the right hepatic lobe from a living donor. N Engl J Med 2002;346:1074–82.

Index

Note: Page numbers of article titles are in **boldface** type.

A

Moving?

Make sure your subscription moves with you!

To notify us of your new address, find your **Clinics Account Number** (located on your mailing label above your name), and contact customer service at:

Email: journalscustomerservice-usa@elsevier.com

800-654-2452 (subscribers in the U.S. & Canada)
314-447-8871 (subscribers outside of the U.S. & Canada)

Fax number: 314-447-8029

Elsevier Health Sciences Division
Subscription Customer Service
3251 Riverport Lane
Maryland Heights, MO 63043

*To ensure uninterrupted delivery of your subscription, please notify us at least 4 weeks in advance of move.

Printed and bound by CPI Group (UK) Ltd, Croydon, CR0 4YY

07/10/2024

01040501-0020